The National
Childbirth
Trust
NCT

Toddler Tantrums

Other titles in this series:

Toddler Tantrums

Penney Hames

Thorsons

An Imprint of HarperCollins*Publishers*

in collaboration with National Childbirth Trust Publishing

To Jane Cleaver, with thanks for
all the shades between black and white

Thorsons/National Childbirth Trust Publishing
Thorsons is an imprint of HarperCollins*Publishers*
77–85 Fulham Palace Road,
Hammersmith, London W6 8JB

The Thorsons website address is:
www.thorsons.com

and *Thorsons*
are trademarks of
HarperCollins*Publishers* Ltd

First published in collaboration
with National Childbirth Trust Publishing 2000
This revised edition published 2002

10 9 8 7 6 5 4

Original photography: Anne Green-Armytage, © 2002 NCT Publishing
Additional photography: Michael Bassett pages 66, 94 and George Williams page 101

Penney Hames asserts the moral right to be
identified as the author of this work

A catalogue record of this book is
available from the British Library

ISBN 0 00 713609 9

Printed and bound in Great Britain by
Martins the Printers Ltd, Berwick upon Tweed

Contents

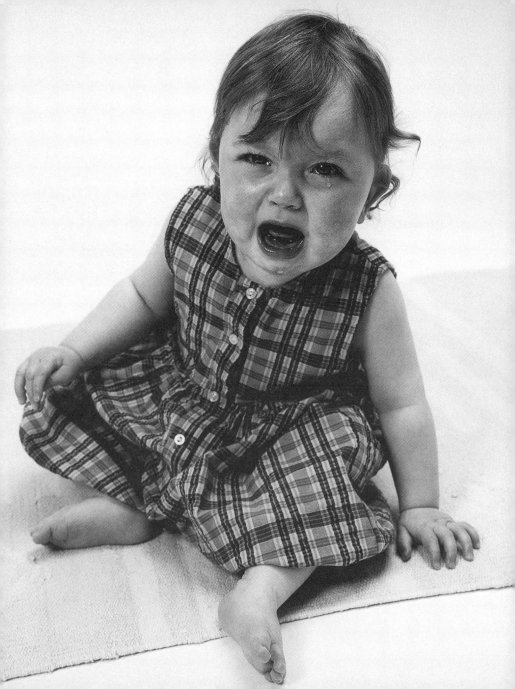

About the Author

Penney Hames, MA, trained first as a journalist and later as a clinical child psychologist. She deferred any practical application of either skill until after a lengthy research and development phase conducted on her own two children, Beany and Richard, and simultaneous years spent writing for the National Childbirth Trust's various national publications on the experiences of parents and babies. She has also written NCT: *Help Your Baby to Sleep* and is co-author of *The NCT Complete Book of Baby Care*. Penney Hames has represented the NCT on the All Party Parliamentary Group on Parenting, and now combines writing with child guidance work in Hampshire.

To laugh often and much; to win the respect of intelligent people and the affection of children; to earn the appreciation of honest critics and endure the betrayal of false friends; to appreciate beauty; to find the best in others; to leave the world a bit better, whether by a healthy child, a garden, or a redeemed social condition; to know even one life has breathed easier because you have lived. This is to have succeeded.

Ralph Waldo Emerson

Acknowledgements

I would like to say thank you to psychologist Dorothy Einon, who generously shared her research results with me in the middle of the marking season, and in between chapters of yet another book. Thank you also to Liz Arbiter of the Tavistock Clinic, who swiftly, surely and repeatedly helped me consider the psychological implications for the toddler who doesn't tantrum. I hope I have done justice to the expertise of both. Any shortcomings or fudges, however, remain undeniably my own responsibility.

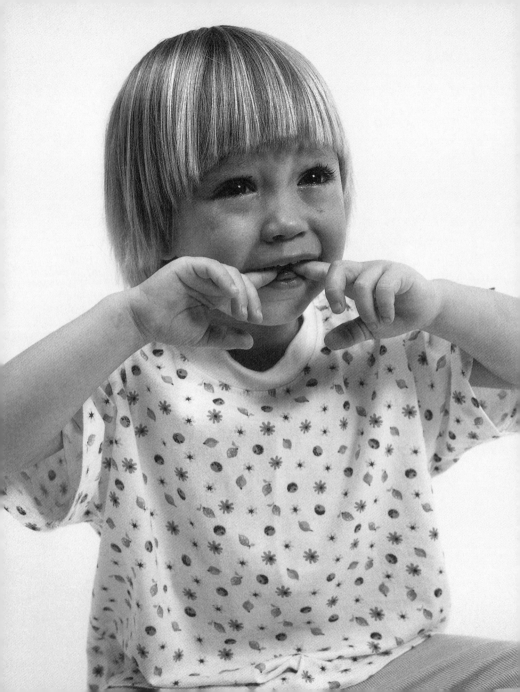

Introduction

A few days ago, I finally looked squarely at something that had been loitering around the edges of my mind for a very long time – maybe since I was a toddler. Why, I wondered, did I find the relationships between parents and children – particularly small children and their new and largely wobbly parents – so endlessly fascinating?

I think it's because I recognize in the toddler–parent relationship a stronger thread of the same uncertainty and repositioning that has woven through my own relationships, not just with my own children, but with my parents and my sisters too.

Toddlers are people in the making and the parents of toddlers are, at the same time, parents in the making. The two processes are irrevocably entwined. New parents with a baby are rapidly learning the basics, but not until they hit toddlerhood do most parents seriously begin to doubt their parenting ability. It's an unsettling time, but this questioning has its virtues. It's not until you question who you are that you can grow up a little. Jostling with our toddlers for space in the family may feel chaotic and uncomfortable, but it gives us the chance to redefine and to deepen our relationship with them and to come to understand ourselves better in the process.

But we don't just create ourselves as parents through our relationships with our toddlers. In becoming the sort of parents we feel good about being, we become more aware of the similarities and differences that we want to make between our own parents and ourselves. In the toddler years, we establish all sorts of limits and boundaries across three generations. And feeling comfortable with this takes time.

Many of the characteristics our toddlers develop and much of our own parenting styles seem to have their roots in the toddler years. In learning to say 'no' firmly but lovingly, and feel good about it, we create space between ourselves and our toddlers that allows them room to flourish in their own way. And leaves us space to develop in ours.

Penney Hames

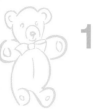

1

What is a Tantrum?

Three-year-old Ruby is standing in the supermarket, her arms locked in position like an angel in a Christmas play, out to her sides, her legs rigid, her eyes wide open and she is screaming. It's a high-pitched, ear-piercing, heart-stopping, agony of a scream. Her mother, hovering nearby, is trying to coax her to 'come on'. Everyone is looking, and even Ruby's mum's friend is shifting uneasily from foot to foot and whispering advice. In the end, Ruby's mum becomes cross and yells at Ruby to 'Stop it immediately.' But Ruby goes on screaming, and by now her face is white, with a blue tinge. Ruby's mum is embarrassed, angry and her bottom lip is quivering. Finally, she picks Ruby up (no mean feat given the rigidity of her daughter's young body) and, abandoning her trolley full of defrosting fish fingers and ice cream in the middle of the aisle, carts her daughter, still screaming, from the supermarket and bundles her into her car seat. Ruby's mum starts the engine and crunches into reverse and away, she doesn't know where, just away. After 15 minutes, Ruby finally stops screaming and falls asleep. Her mother is exhausted, confused and the first of many tears runs down her cheek.

A tantrum is a supercharged emotional explosion that occurs when your toddler feels out of control. It's a practical demonstration of how your toddler feels inside – chaotic, confused and in pieces. Almost all tantrums happen when your toddler is with the people that she loves the most – which probably means you. But then you knew it was tough being a parent.

But tantrums are more than just shows of temper. Temper may be how it looks to you. In a temper may be how it makes you feel. But if you think of them as 'temper tantrums', and nothing more, you are not only doing your toddler a disservice, but you may also waste one of the most valuable opportunities you will ever have for helping your toddler come to terms with strong emotions.

In one sense, tantrums are natural, frequent and, believe it or not, positive steps forward in your child's development. Tantrums prove that your toddler is beginning to develop a sense of herself, and a sense of her place in the world. Throwing a tantrum is your toddler's way of coping with the frustration that she feels when she can't hang on any longer to her fragile sense of who she is, and how she fits in.

Toddlers begin to learn where they end and others begin in two ways:

- by doing things
- through their relationship with you

Busy Doing Nothing

Toddlers are busy people for good reason. A toddler's sense of herself is bound up with doing things. When you are two or three, activity is the best way to work out who you are – pretending, digging, incessantly chatting, taking things apart, running, climbing, sorting, shouting – all are activities that provide your toddler with a firmer sense of herself.

It's by *doing* that toddlers discover their strengths and weaknesses. And it's by *choosing* what they do (within limits) that toddlers discover their likes and dislikes – they discover themselves. Toddlers need plenty to do and lots of (limited) choice.

If you have to say 'no' to your toddler, offer him two other choices, so that he can still feel in control. Choices give your toddler the chance to escape with dignity.

Two-year-old Charlie began to stroke Jonathan's curls with a wooden hammer, but Mike, Charlie's dad, stepped in before Charlie thought of another use for his toy. 'Here Charlie, let's swop,' he said. 'Which would you prefer – this comb or this little red brush?' Charlie happily dropped the hammer.

But toddlers aren't able to limit what they want, at least not at first. A young toddler's only concern is to do what she wants and to do it NOW. So, when you say 'no' to your toddler, or even ask her to wait, she doesn't have the brainpower to coolly consider your point of view – she doesn't even yet realize you have a point of view. All she feels is confused and incredibly frustrated.

Toddlers are spontaneous individuals for whom a second is a long time and a minute an impossibility. For toddlers there is only now. They can't think about later. They can't imagine five minutes' time, let alone tomorrow afternoon. Your toddler's frustration is born out of a desire to do whatever it is she has in mind immediately.

Frustration generates a lot of tension which has to be expressed somehow, and hurling yourself to the floor, thrashing wildly and screaming as loud as you can is a magnificent way of releasing that tension immediately.

The sort of things that will frustrate your toddler are:

- not being given what she wants – your attention, more sweets, *that* toy
- not being able to do things herself – getting dressed (socks are a particular tantrum trigger), carry all her toys at once, cross the road without holding your hand

- wanting you to do something that you can't or won't do – such as allowing her to choose your groceries, stay with her while she falls asleep
- not knowing what she wants – to eat her tea at the table or to sit on the sofa with Granddad, and miss tea
- not being able to explain what she wants – that she wants to go higher but not faster on the swing, for example. (OK, that's impossible, but she doesn't know that and it doesn't stop her frustration)
- not being able to control everything – including the colour of her sandwich plate and you. This is one reason why imaginative play is so important at this age – it allows your toddler complete control
- being misunderstood – which includes being laughed at when she hadn't meant to be funny
- boredom
- tiredness
- hunger
- illness

Any of these things can stop your toddler in her tracks and trigger a tantrum.

Tantrum-free Toddlers

Of course, some parents say that their toddlers just don't tantrum. And this makes sense because there is enormous variability amongst toddlers just as there is enormous variability amongst the families in which toddlers live. However, it may be that some toddlers do tantrum, but their tantrums are not recognized. One parent's tantrum is another parent's protest. So, two toddlers may do exactly the same things, but one set of parents will say that their toddler threw a tantrum and the other that their toddler got a bit cross. In some families, admitting to tantrums may feel like failure. But it may be more helpful to think about tantrums another way. The truth is that weathering a tantrum can teach our toddlers and ourselves how we fit together.

Expressing Emotions

Naturally, there are a few toddlers who just don't tantrum. Sometimes, entire families of children pass through their toddler years without ever throwing a wobbly. And in other families, some toddlers tantrum and others don't. The reason for this is unclear and unresearched. Perhaps the less demonstrative siblings are allowing the noisier ones to shout and scream on their behalf.

It's also possible that toddlers who don't tantrum were babies who were quickly shushed every time they cried, because their parents couldn't bear to hear their sadness. If we haven't learnt to deal with our own sadness, it is very difficult to help our babies and toddlers to deal with theirs. And the same goes for frustration and anger, success and happiness. The better we are at recognizing these emotions in ourselves, the more at ease we'll be when our toddlers feel them too.

Toddlers who don't tantrum may already sense that great displays of emotion are not comfortable for their family. If a toddler knows that her parents find anger and frustration difficult then she may decide it's safer to deal with these emotions in a different way. Being obstinate, stubborn, highly verbal, deliberately slow, endlessly active or – what is really unusual in a toddler – just waiting, are all ways for your toddler to maintain self-control and avoid a full-blown tantrum.

Toddlers adapt their behaviour to match ours. Parents who go in for explosive bursts of temper will probably have toddlers who enjoy exploding too. Careful, controlled parents are likely to have careful, controlled toddlers.

One thing I have found, however, is that toddlers who don't tantrum tend to be socially different from toddlers who do. Non-tantrummers like to keep themselves to themselves. They prefer to stand back from the hurly-burly of toddler life and let others go first. Oliver, at 26 months, has never tantrummed. He lets all the other children go first when the box of musical instruments is put out at nursery. If there's nothing left for him then he's quite happy just to sing. At least he hasn't had to push in to get his way.

It seems to be a common and long-lasting pattern. Suzy, now nearly seven years old, never had a tantrum when she was little. Now, at the top of the infant school she is quiet in groups, and anxious whenever she has to change for PE. Maybe this is because she feels exposed when she undresses in front of others, but it's just as likely to be her way of stubbornly maintaining control.

Non-tantrummers have the sort of self-control that seems to continue into later childhood in the form of stubbornness or anxiety, and the need for reassurance and explanations. On the other hand, non-tantrummers also seem to have good verbal skills, to be more patient, and more confident once they know the score. Isabel, another non-tantrummer who is now five, became potty-trained very late, but completed it in an afternoon. She did the same with walking. Non-tantrummers are often more easy-going playmates too because they make it their business to adapt to the needs of the other child.

The important thing to ensure is that your toddler's needs and wishes are respected. You don't have to agree to everything she wants, but it's good to acknowledge that her wishes exist. 'You want to stay in the park; you're having a lovely time, but we must go home now', is better than, 'We're going home now', because it acknowledges your toddler's feelings and shows that you can cope with the anger, frustration and sadness that she expresses. These powerful emotions need to be accepted, acknowledged and dealt with so that your toddler will one day be able to manage the bigger angers and frustrations of later life.

If you find it hard to allow your toddler to be unhappy or frustrated take a look at Chapter 8 for some suggestions.

Your Toddler's Relationship with You

Your toddler's relationship with you can also cause her to tantrum because she has yet to accept easily where she ends and you begin. Little by little over the past year and a half she has been coming to terms with the idea that you and she are not one and the same person. Now, at 18 months, give or take a month or two, she finally accepts that truth. She is, by turns, delighted with the freedom this gives her and horrified by the lack of security. At one and the same time she asserts her right to do whatever she decides to do and yet to have you with her emotionally every inch of the way.

She may no longer need you to feed, dress and fetch toys for her, as much as you once did, but she still needs you to love her, comfort her and protect her from herself. When she was a baby, she needed you to order her day – to lay her down when she was ready for sleep, feed her when she was hungry, change her nappy when she was uncomfortable. Now, as a toddler, she needs you to order her mind as well – to use actions and words to make sense of what she feels and thinks.

The most important way that you do this is by giving your toddler your attention. The more attention your toddler gets, the more she understands herself, and the more she understands herself, the happier she is. For your toddler, attention equals love. But if you're busy looking after the baby, working to pay the mortgage, cleaning, cooking and generally doing, your toddler may get to feel a little unloved.

Toddlers soon learn the best ways to get your attention – sitting on your lap, hanging on to your ankle as you make lunch, drawing on the wall, weeing on the carpet, raiding the fridge, deadheading all the flowers that are still in full bloom, hugging the baby lovingly round the neck, walking through big brother's Lego model. Toddlers who feel ignored grab your attention in any way they can. To put it bluntly, tantrums occur more when you have less time to pay attention to your toddler.

By becoming a mirror in which your toddler can see herself, you provide her with a picture of herself. She needs you to be there and involved with her in order to make sense of herself. Which is why 99 per cent of tantrums occur when you are with your toddler but unable to give her your full attention. Talking on the phone and shopping are only the two most obvious scenarios – cooking tea, the entire run-up to Christmas, and packing for a holiday can be just as bad. She's got you there, right in front of her, but she just can't seem to get you to concentrate. It's not that toddlers want to be the centre of attention – they're not clever enough for that – it's that they lose track of themselves when nobody is focusing on them. And the younger the toddler, the more attention she needs to stay happy.

Older toddlers are often pretty good at expressing themselves, which can make their tantrums even more annoying. But frustration can tie tongues. Your toddler may need you to help her understand what she's feeling. If you can describe what's going on for your toddler it may help her to stay calm.

If you find it hard to imagine what your toddler is feeling try tuning into what you're feeling and describe that to her as though it were what she was feeling – when emotions are running high, they are amazingly contagious.

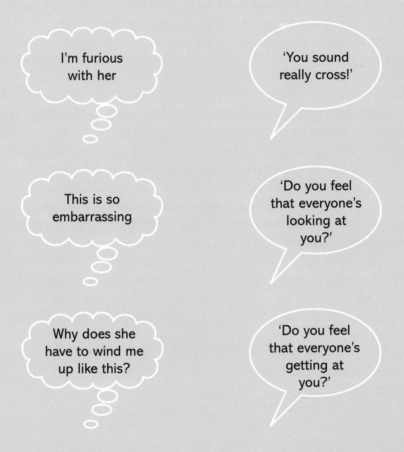

Even if you don't hit the nail right on the head every time, she'll appreciate that you are trying to understand her.

Try thinking of your toddler as a stream flowing swiftly between the banks of your parenting. If you stop her mid-flow by asking her to wait a minute, she can't just wait patiently – there is the whole river coming down behind her, pushing her inexorably on, adding ever more and more pressure to her need to move forward. The river needs to come out, to express itself, but there is no place to go once the way ahead is dammed. The result is a chaotic circling, a rushing to and fro on the spot, a search for an escape route (this is where the tantrum begins – your toddler is still standing but stamping her feet and drumming her arms). Ultimately there is an eruption, a flooding over the banks that normally hold the river to its course (your toddler flings herself to the floor, and screams and drums her heels, her arms and maybe her head as well). When they have finally finished gushing, the flood waters need careful handling. They need scooping up and reincorporating in the river, and the banks need to be rebuilt (you offer a cuddle to your contrite and maybe still-sobbing toddler and you let her know that even though you didn't accept her behaviour you still love her, and then you make sure you award yourself some brownie points and have a few minutes to yourself as soon as you can).

Of course, it's something your toddler needs to learn how to do – cope without you. But a tantrum, at least while your toddler is under about two and a half, is a loud and clear message that she can't cope right now.

But, just because tantrums are understandable, doesn't mean they are acceptable. You need to let your toddler know that:

- tantrums are an unacceptable way of communicating
- there are other ways that she can let you know she wants you
- you believe she will learn other ways in time

Age Differences

Tantrums at 18 months differ from tantrums at three years. This is because, by three, your toddler will have a better memory, more developed social skills, a clearer sense of who she is, more control over her behaviour, and if you've been saying it loud and clear, she will have got the message that tantrums are unacceptable.

At 18 months, most toddlers have between two tantrums a day and three a week. A few have none, while a few others have as many (and sometimes more than) five a day. The average length is about three minutes from start to finish, although some toddlers have a lot more sticking power.

At 18 months, a tantrum ends as suddenly as it begins, and lasts for about three minutes. There are two stages to these tantrums:

- your toddler gives you the 'reason' for the tantrum
- the physical performance of the tantrum

Toddlers of this age can be divided into two groups:

- droppers: who drop to the floor at your feet, yelling, screaming, drumming their heels and their arms
- separators: who push you away or run away themselves, sometimes using their legs to kick out at you as well

The significant thing is that neither group moves completely out of your sight – these tantrums are about your relationship with her, so there is no way that your toddler wants to lose sight of you completely. Because they come and go so quickly, these tantrums are easier to laugh at. Toddlers of this age seem to collapse into a tantrum – with little or no control over the stopping or the starting of them.

Once the immediate tantrum is over, it is almost as if nothing has happened. Certainly your toddler is often smiling and skipping within minutes of a tantrum. Fortunately, because it's all so quick, you may feel the same, and once the tantrum is over, you often both forget it.

As toddlers get older, additional stages are added. Tantrums now have a beginning, a middle and an end, and last that bit longer. Some toddlers of this age have the ability to string a tantrum out for an hour or so:

- Pre-drama stage: niggling, mumbling, spoiling for a fight. Your toddler may mutter something followed by 'You do it'. If you then ask 'What?' she has the perfect excuse (as far as she's concerned) to tantrum. At this stage tantrums are predictable, but with swift and decisive action you can sometimes prevent them. (There are a few suggestions to try in Chapter 3.)
- Standing-up stage: drumming of arms and legs, screaming, shouting.
- Falling-on-the-floor stage: arches back, kicks legs, some toddlers bang their heads against the floor or the wall raising great bruises and a few bite their arms until they bleed. At this age self-harming does not necessarily indicate deep psychological trauma. Although you may well be psychologically traumatized by watching it.
- Sad-and-sorry stage: screams turn to whimpers and sobs; she knows she has behaved appallingly. Some toddlers will allow you to comfort them, others will stand next to you but don't want to be held. Your toddler is subdued.

These tantrums are more difficult to ignore, make you feel more wound up and take both of you longer to recover from. By this age, your toddler knows she can get an effect by behaving in this way (she is truly 'throwing' the tantrum), but she is still out of control when she's going through it. It's this loss of control that makes her scared and sorry once the shouting is over.

Many toddlers outgrow tantrums by the time they are four or so, although many others go on having the occasional one for many years. A small number of children still have regular tantrums at four and a half and they fall into two groups:

- those who started early – before 18 months – and are now having tantrums that are longer, more frequent and may involve hurting others and breaking things
- those who started later – around three years, maybe as a response to the birth of a sibling – and are now having milder, less frequent tantrums

Both groups are more likely to bang things rather than fall on the floor by now.

In the beginning, no toddler is in control of the feelings of outrage and frustration that spin her into a tantrum. But as she grows you may notice telltale signs that your toddler has learnt that tantrumming gets her what she wants, quicker than she can say 'please' and 'thank you':

- there's a build-up to the tantrum – mumbling, shuffling, spoiling for a fight
- following you from room to room and lying down at your feet each time
- only throwing a wobbly when other people are around
- stopping and starting depending on whether or not you are looking.
- lifting her head to see whether you are still watching or whether she should give it up and join in again

> Eliott was just two years old and he was tantrumming in the kitchen. I can't even remember what for, I think I'd given him the wrong cup, or something. He was lying on the floor screaming and kicking and I walked out of the room and ignored him. And then, blow me, he got up and followed me into the lounge. It was at that point I knew that I could call his bluff. And after that I just ignored his tantrums and they faded away.

Alison, mother of Eliott, now seven

None of this means that your child is scheming, but just that she has learnt what works for her. If she didn't do what she knows works she wouldn't be human.

Why do Toddlers Go on Tantrumming?

Because there's always the chance it will get them what they want. Most of the time this 'something' is one of two things:

- your attention
- a particular thing: more sweets/another turn on the see-saw/no bath

The chances are that, like the rest of us, you or your partner gave in once or twice when your toddler threw a tantrum and now she believes that all she has to do is hold out for long enough and she'll get what she wants. Don't give her your attention and don't give her what she screams for. (Try Chapter 5 for the most effective ways to do this.) She needs to learn:

- that tantrums don't work
- some alternative routes to getting what she wants. (There are some good ideas about doing this in Chapter 8.)

2

How to Have
Fewer Tantrums

The other day, Rachel, a young mum I've known for a long time, tele-phoned. 'I've got myself into a right state,' she said, 'and I don't know what to do.' I listened as she continued: 'I've been a lot firmer than usual with Ben and Emily over the last two weeks and it really seems to have paid off in terms of their behaviour. Initially, they were really stroppy about it but by last Wednesday they seemed to sense that "Mummy now meant what she said" and somehow they seemed much happier in them-selves. And we've definitely had fewer tantrums than before. But then they went to stay with Michael's mum and now they're really playing up again and they seem a lot less happy than before the weekend.'

Rachel continued to talk and explained that her mother-in-law had deliberately flouted two of her new rules: 'no sweets before tea' and 'no jumping on the beds'. Her mother-in-law, it seems, had felt that the new rules were a bit hard for little tots and had given in to the twins' demands, asking them to keep the sweets and the jumps as a secret: 'Just the three of us. Just this once.' But the twins had been unable to keep quiet. In fact, Emily had been very worried about keeping such a naughty secret, and didn't want Rachel to be cross.

By the time we'd finished talking, Rachel sounded calmer and she had made up her mind to have a quiet chat with her mother-in-law. It was either that or the twins would have to give up seeing her for a while.

What this story tells us, I think, is that toddlers feel happier when the adults around them are firm, fair and predictable. Toddlers may kick up a fuss if they don't get what they want, but they prefer that to never knowing where they stand. Toddlers like and respect adults who can say 'no' as well as 'yes'.

You can avoid some tantrums by tuning into what your toddlers need, rather than to what they say they want.

There is no foolproof way to avoid toddler tantrums altogether. It's hard, but there it is. In fact, some experts believe that it would be wrong to try. Tantrums, they say, are an essential part of growing up, and the toddler who doesn't tantrum misses out on a valuable experience. On the other hand, there are also experts who say that if you come down hard on your toddler the first time he tantrums you won't have many other tantrums to deal with. I'm not sure I go along with either of these. What I am sure of, though, is that tantrums are such a common part of being a toddler that most parents will have to weather some.

But that doesn't mean there's nothing you can do. You can reduce the number of tantrums by listening hard to what your toddler is saying. Toddlers (like the rest of us) are happier, and less ready to tantrum, when they know where they stand and they feel OK about it. So, how do you manage this? I think it depends on the balance of three things:

- needs
- wants
- expectations

Needs, Wants ...

Your toddler is busy trying to find out where he fits in and what he's allowed to do. He doesn't want to be a baby any more, but he's not mature or clever enough to be a child either. So, how does he find out what his place is in your family? How does he discover exactly how far he can go? Basically, he tries anything once. In watching you and other children he will get an idea of the sorts of things people do and then he will set out to do them. He's a great imitator. And as far as he's concerned once he can do all the things you do, he will be a grown-up. Sally and Jo both find this an exhausting time, and have worked out their own solutions to the problem. Sally first:

> She's been going through this stage of wanting to help me all the time. And I'm getting to the point where I feel she's all over me all the time. Last week I gave her a duster so she could help me polish and shine, and I had a duster too and a can of spray. But she kept trying to take the spray polish off me and I kept putting a little bit of the polish on her duster and I kept saying "No, let Mummy do this."
>
> Well in the end she threw a real wobbly. She threw herself on the bed and cried and screamed, for about two minutes. But I'd said "no" because her safety was paramount in my mind – she could have sprayed it anywhere. There was no way she could have had it. In the end I coaxed her out of it and found her something else to do. I distracted her attention. And gave her a hug. I told her that the polish was dangerous but I had a new job for her. I made her feel that putting all the knick-knacks on to the bed was just as important.

Sally, mother of Abbie, two

> Elliot has difficulty following instructions to either hold my hand or sit in the buggy whilst out on the roads. I understand that he wants to walk now he's a "big boy" but he is prone to running-walking and not stopping even if I shout my loudest at him. If I tell him to get in the buggy he screams at me a loud "no" and there is no way I can physically cajole him. So I give him two options: "Hold the buggy or my/your brother's hand." This works immediately 40 per cent of the time but the rest of the time he replies with a determined "no". Then I'll try: "Well, help Mummy to push the buggy then." This works in the majority of cases but he has been known to refuse even this. At this point if it's a short walk I'll carry him or if a long one I'll strap him into the seat promising to do something – "Let's go see the trains/pop into the pet shop/go to the baker's ..." etc. This one always works but it's my last port of call.

Jo, mother of Elliot, two and a half

Your toddler has no conception of what it would feel like inside to be a grown-up. He only sees the outside bits – driving the car, chopping salad, polishing windows – and he wants to do those things too. He pushes at the limits all the time – demanding to do more and more of the things he wants, more and more of the things that he sees you doing, or other children doing. It's only when you say 'no' firmly and calmly that he learns where he stops and adults begin. He learns that there is more to being big than just doing the things that big people do, although you may have to weather many tantrums before he accepts this fact.

'Benjamin doesn't tantrum in typical fashion – I mean he doesn't throw himself on the floor. But he knows exactly what he thinks is sensible to do. And he's furious if he's not allowed to do everything that the adults do. Yesterday he said "I'm just going to post these letters up the road, Mummy." Obviously, I insisted that he wasn't going to do it. So he screamed for about 30 seconds. This happens on many, many occasions. He is constantly striving for independence. He runs his own bath, gets his own drink and dresses himself, and he can do his own breakfast, and his sister's, which is great. But now he wants to drive the car, he wants to wash up and he wants to choose his food – and if we don't allow him he gives us a 30-second scream. On a bad day he might scream 50 times a day, on a good day, only five.

When I'm irritated or we can't divert him or he's screaming too much I feel the best place is upstairs and I take him to his room and say "Come down when you are going to be more reasonable." On a bad day he goes to his room four or five times a day. Each time he struggles and fights when he is put there, but he's always down quickly – often within a few seconds and it's all forgotten.'

Mandy, mother of Benjamin, three

But when is it reasonable to say 'no'? How can we help our toddlers to go on feeling good about the things they can do without letting the illusion of being grown-up take over? It's a difficult balancing trick. This is where it's useful to think about the difference between wants and needs. Briefly, your toddler needs to be allowed to do (or to have) the things he needs, but he (like everyone else) should have only some of the things he wants.

So let's just remind ourselves what the difference is. Needs are things like:

- food, water, love
- shelter, being listened to
- freedom from fear of harm
- having someone attempt to understand you
- having limits
- time alone ...

... and plenty of other things too. Basically, needs amount to being treated like a human being, not a possession or an extension of another person or a pet. It's only when we feel that our needs are met that we can start to enjoy life ... and think about what we want.

Personally, I want three-day weekends, longer summers and a self-cleaning house. Your toddler's wants will be different – and much more immediate. Toddlers always want things right now. He may ask to sit on your lap at teatime, to stay up until you go to bed, to open and investigate the contents of your bag or pockets, or to be first to eat the new cereal. You will have to decide which of these is fair and reasonable and which it is reasonable to refuse. Wants are those things which define us as individuals. Being given something of what we want allows us to become the person we want to be – within limits. A little bit of what you fancy does you good.

Recently, American researchers discovered that children who are given sweets by their parents are better able to regulate how many sweets they eat at other times. In an experiment, toddlers who were normally given sweets now and again were compared to children whose parents never allowed them sweets. The two groups of children were given unlimited sweets by the investigators. The children who had sweets now and again ate some and then stopped. The children who never had any kept on eating and eating.

Simply put, toddlers who aren't allowed to practise having a little of what they want never learn when they have had enough.

So why is it so hard to get this right? Two reasons, I think:

1 We Don't Like to be Mean

When your toddler was a small, but perfectly gorgeous, bundle of a baby, he couldn't do anything for himself. He needed help with eating, drinking, dressing ... well, pretty much everything, really. It was easy to tell when he needed something because he would cry. You might not always have known what it was he needed, but that's a different story. The fact was that your baby had nothing but needs. He needed to sleep, he needed to feed, he needed to be played with ... and so on. And even though this was exhausting at times, there was one good thing about a baby's needs – you never had to decide whether to do anything about them – the answer was always 'yes'. Needs have to be met.

Your toddler, on the other hand, has discovered wants. Big time. He wants to eat his pudding before his savoury ... he wants to stay and play when you need to go home ... he wants to dig the garden ... he wants your friends to go home so you will play with him. And only some of these will be reasonable, some of the time. But our toddlers have a knack of making us feel that we are mean to say 'no' because they believe, without a shadow of a doubt, that whatever they want, they need. In this respect at least, your toddler still wants you to treat him like the baby he once was. He wants you to give him everything he wants. But if you do, he will stay like a demanding baby for far too long. In fact, far from being mean to say 'no', you would be mean to say 'yes' all the time, because you wouldn't give him the chance to grow up. Caroline has found it works for her:

I've discovered that if I draw a line and say "No, I'm not going beyond this", it actually works. He had a paddy the other day about his tea. He refused to eat it but he wanted the pudding. Well, I said "I do love you very much but I'm afraid if you don't eat that food, you're not having a pudding." Well, he cried and he cried and he cried and it was awful. But then he finally realized that I did mean business and said "Will you heat this up again Mummy, please?" and I did and he ate it – quite reasonable after all. And then later the next day I heard him say, during a game with his sister, Lydia, "Mummy says if you don't eat that food you are not having a pudding." He'd learnt the rule and I thought, "Oh well, it was actually worth that hassle." He hasn't held it against me.

Caroline, mother of Isaac, four

I remember a small cousin of mine toddling up to my mum and saying that she 'needed an apple'. For her, any want *was* a need. For other toddlers it's the other way round. All their needs *sound like* wants. 'I want a cuddle ...' 'I want a story ...' 'I want to finish this puzzle before bed ...' And maybe some of these, some of the time, are really needs. Toddlers aren't clear about this, so it's doubly important that we are.

What Your Toddler Needs

When you ask your pre-tantrum toddler what the matter is he may say 'I want that toy' or 'I want a drink'. What he may mean, however, is that he is bored. When he says 'I want to go first' or 'I don't want to go in my buggy', what he may mean is that he is tired. When your toddler says he *wants* X, Y or Z, he may be telling you that he *needs* A, B or C. When you're having difficulty understanding what he really needs, chances are he is too.

When you're confused stop and think.

- What is he really saying?
- Is he tired, hungry, thirsty, bored, feeling ignored or unimportant ...?
- How can I give him what he really needs?

If you think you can see what your toddler really needs, try to help him out. If he's bored, can you stop what you are doing and do something else? If he is tired, can you offer him a five-minute cuddle? Tell him what need you are meeting. When he deliberately removes all the CDs from the rack when you have company: 'You're feeling left out aren't you – would you like to come and sit with me?' When he starts to throw the toys in the overheated waiting room at the doctor's: 'This room is very stuffy, let's take our sweatshirts off.' But gently does it. Keep it subtle. Toddlers learn quickly to deny that they are tired, so if tiredness is the root cause don't point this out. That's too much like an admission of failure for an active toddler!

What is very sad, though, is the toddler who learns that sometimes his *needs* don't get met. Needs, like those in the list on page 20, are not optional extras. They need to be freely provided. Toddlers who frequently don't have their needs met learn to cope in one of three ways:

- They learn to ask indirectly. Toddlers who whine or lie or are exceedingly timid or good may feel that this is the only way they can get what they need.
- They learn to ask through actions. Toddlers who tantrum at the smallest thing, or for hours on end, or are repeatedly naughty or aggressive may be trying to get what they need.
- They learn to deny that they have particular needs at all, and eventually to deny these same needs in others. Toddlers who break away from cuddles, or who never cry, may have lost touch with their own needs.

Of course, all toddlers whine and all toddlers are naughty, but if your toddler seems to do nothing else then maybe you will need to do some hard thinking about what he might be trying to say. Chapter 7 may help you to strike a balance that feels right.

Toddlers often seem to tantrum over the smallest things – the colour of a balloon, the shape of their sandwiches, the way that you have drawn a picture – things that, to an adult, seem trivial. 'I want the yellow one/triangles/a different cat.' Sometimes these things are amazingly important to your toddler and it may be worth trying to see why from his perspective some of the time, like Jane:

> We lived in America for a couple of years and one day we were in a church and it was time for coffee and Charlotte decided that she wanted to run up and down. Well that was OK for a while, but then we said it was time to go. She protested, I think there was a particular run that she wanted to do, but we said, "You've had plenty of time" and we put her in the car. But as we went off down the road she got worse and worse and in the end we decided we had to go back. By the time we managed to drive back they'd locked the church but there was a car park and we said, "Would you like to race here?" Luckily she did. Then she got back in the car and was as right as rain. I think the moral of the story is that sometimes, if there's something a child really, really wants to do, it's worth letting them do it. So long as it doesn't inconvenience you and it isn't dangerous, it can be worth letting them go with the flow. Sometimes you have to see the importance through the eyes of the child.

Jane, mother of Charlotte, aged two and a half

A toddler who feels he is being given what he wants, at least some of the time, will become more reasonable about those times that you just cannot fall in with his wishes, as Ruth has found:

One day Callum asked for ham sandwiches for lunch. I made them, cut the crusts off, just as he likes, and gave them to him. He took one look and wailed, flinging his arms down on the table with a comment like "I didn't want them like ..." His speech became absorbed in hysterics and I never heard the rest. At first I responded with "Well, you asked for ham. I might just take them away again." His wails became sobs and he flung his body to the floor. I couldn't understand what I had done that was so distressing – only a ham sandwich after all. A good 10 minutes went by before he calmed down. Then I suggested that a different sandwich was what he wanted. It took a while before he could speak. In the end he said the ham was fine but he wanted squares not triangles!

Since then there have been many of these. Now I try to pre-empt any complaints by finding out exactly what he wants, how he wants it and take time to explain in full and in advance if I cannot achieve his objectives. The worst thing anyone can do is laugh at his specific requests and language, attempt to tickle him out of it or give unwanted physical comfort.

Ruth, mother of Callum, four and a half

The Pooh Bear Paddy

Have you noticed how often your toddler yells for some particular thing and then, having been given it, immediately demands something else? 'I want that hammer' (that Peter has) your toddler shouts. You give him an exact replica (pleased that you can solve this so simply), but he continues to reach out and whine for the one that Peter has. You and Peter's father eventually agree to swop the hammers, but no sooner have you done so than your toddler demands that you give him back the one he first had. Many toddlers find it hard to choose between two things they want. Rather like Pooh, who, on being asked by Rabbit whether he would prefer honey or condensed milk with his bread, said 'Both.'

Your toddler also wants both. But 'both' is unreasonable, where a second child is involved. The only thing to do is to stand firm and let your toddler experience and live through the frustration, as Margaret did:

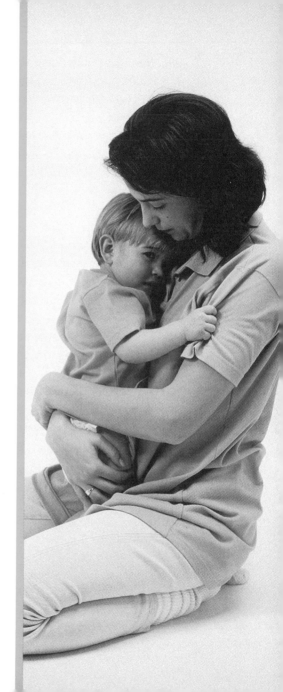

Kathleen gave a balloon she had been playing with at the childminder's to Thomas, another boy who is looked after there, and I said "That's very nice of you." But just at the last minute she wanted to take the balloon home with her. "Ah … you've just given it to Thomas. You can't have it back." Well she threw herself on the floor and cried and cried and both the childminder and I tried to console her, but she was beside herself. In the end her childminder said she could have another balloon, and went off to get one. But this was no good – she still wanted the old balloon, so we swopped the two over – Thomas was really too little to mind – but then she wanted the new balloon.

At that point I said "This is outrageous" and we went home with her still screaming, and no balloons. She recovered after about 10 minutes in the car – after I had tried turning the music on. (She'd said, "Turn the music off, mummy.") I asked her if she would talk. (She said, "No.") I asked her if she would be quiet. (She carried on screaming.) And then I tried shouting – but that never works. When she finally quietened down, I stopped the car and we talked about the day and came round to the balloons. She got the message that it was because she tantrummed that she didn't get either. We talked about sharing. It was a tough one. With Kathleen, if you give her choices, you get yourself into deep water. She just can't decide.

Margaret, mother of Kathleen, two and a half

Margaret stood firm about Kathleen's demand for both balloons. The only thing that might have been even more effective was Margaret's silence until Kathleen was ready to talk. Sometimes it's hard to let our toddlers work through their frustration on their own. But until they do it's almost impossible to suggest anything that will be right.

If your toddler is going through the Pooh Bear stage you can give him practice with no-lose choices. Choices like:

- 'Do you want to go on the swings or the slide first?'
- 'Which sweetie are you going to eat now and which are you going to save for after tea?'
- 'Shall we cycle to Alan's house through the park, and then come back past the shops, or shall we go past the shops on the way there?'

But if any choice makes him anxious, decide for him for a while:

- 'Here are your clothes.'
- 'Here is your bowl of cereal.'
- 'You can have a few crisps now and I'll save the rest for later.'

Later, he'll be able to cope with more decisions.

Life without some of our wants being met would be a dull affair, but a life where every little want is met is a life of tyranny and despair. Tyranny because the toddler who shouts or whines until he gets what he wants feels that he has control, and despair because in gaining control he has lost something much more precious – the unbounded love of his parents. Toddlers, like the rest of us, are happier when they are given what they need, than when they are given what they whine for.

In fact, if you look back at the list of needs on page 20 you'll see that limits are a basic need. We all need limits. Limits help us to feel safe and secure. So in saying 'no' to some of the things that your toddler demands you are in fact meeting one of his needs – a much more important achievement.

... and Expectations

But needs and wants are not the full story. From the first few weeks of life babies start to make connections between things. 'If I cry then someone comes.' 'If I smile then someone smiles back.' They are learning what to expect; they are learning that they can have an effect. By now your toddler has developed some pretty sophisticated expectations of all sorts of things.

Your toddler is clever. Already he expects you to say 'no' to certain things: he expects you to say 'no' to dangerous things like taking the cakes from the oven. He expects you to say 'no' to hurtful things like pushing other children. He expects you to say 'no' to annoying things like faffing around when it's time to get dressed. On the other hand, he expects you to say 'yes' when he asks to do helpful things like lay the table, 'yes' when he wants to do heart-warming things like give you a hug and 'yes' when he wants to do creative things like dance round the living room.

But there are, of course, many other things where the answer will sometimes be 'yes' and sometimes 'no'. Things like pouring a drink or making mud pies, or calling grandma on the phone. Which means that it's more difficult for your toddler to know what to expect from you.

What toddlers need in these sorts of situations is as much certainty as possible. The best thing that you can do is to stick to what you say. Say 'yes' or say 'no' and then don't budge. If he sees once that he can change your mind by whining, crying, shouting or screaming your clever toddler will almost certainly try the same tactics next time.

He will have learnt that he can't expect you to behave in a consistent way. He will also have learnt that he can be more powerful than you. But neither of these are comfortable lessons for a toddler. When you give in to your toddler's protests, toddlers can feel frightened by their power, and far from being happy, may continue to whine because their need for limits have not been met.

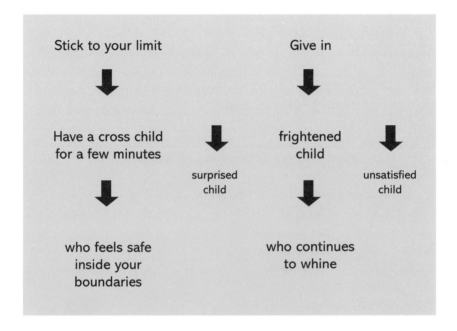

Stick to your limit   Give in

Have a cross child   frightened
for a few minutes   child

      surprised   unsatisfied
      child   child

who feels safe   who continues
inside your   to whine
boundaries

Toddlers like to know what to expect. Even when they expect something that they don't want they still prefer it to having their need for safe limits ignored.

But old habits die hard. Once you decide never to give in again to an unreasonable demand or a tantrum, be prepared to meet a lot of resistance. Expect your toddler to keep on demanding for a long time. He was used to the old pattern, and even though it made him feel insecure or unhappy, he still wants it because that is what he knows. Stand firm, stay calm and you can help him to get used to being cross but happy. A kinder sort of parenting.

But expectations work the other way round too. Toddlers don't just expect us to behave in certain ways, they know that *we* expect *them* to behave in certain ways too. Most of the time, toddlers try their hardest to please us. To fit in with what they think we expect. The truth is that if you expect the worst, you'll get it. But if you let your toddler know that you expect better, you'll get that instead. Of course, none of us says 'Now Peter, I expect you to be as naughty as you can at Auntie Elaine's.' The messages we give are a little more subtle than that. A raised eyebrow or a sigh, for example, can say 'Oh, not again. I should have known ...' more eloquently than any number of fine words.

This is why it's better to say:

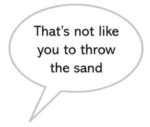

That's not like
you to throw
the sand

Even if he often does throw the sand. Rather than:

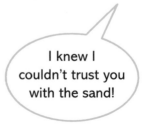

I knew I
couldn't trust you
with the sand!

And:

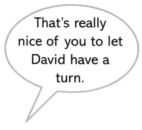

as he is momentarily distracted from hogging the slide for himself by the offer of a biscuit, rather than:

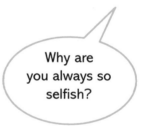

Your toddler will try to rise to those expectations you have of him.

Consistency

The more consistent you are, the easier it will be for your toddler to learn what to expect, and to feel safe about how he fits in with everyone around him.

Sam has learnt the hard way to be consistent about Rory's tantrums:

> Rory sometimes wakes in a really grouchy mood from his afternoon snooze. He arches his back, hits out and screams. Putting him on the floor makes him worse, but picking him up is painful! So I put him down, walk away and ignore him. The cries of "Mama!" are heart-rending, but as soon as I approach he rejects me and refuses to be picked up. (On one occasion I had an acquaintance round; she watched him go through this and she clearly wanted me to pick him up. I demonstrated twice what happened when I tried, so we carried on chatting together and ignoring him! After a few minutes more, the screams turned to sobbing; I opened my arms to Rory and asked him for a cuddle and he came to me; all was then well in his little world.) I hope I am communicating that I am always there if he wants me, but there is some behaviour I will not accept, and he can come and find me when he has calmed down.

Sam, mother of Rory, 20 months

A consistent approach may often sound like a broken record. And that's fine. For example, if you don't want your toddler to climb on the table you will have to say 'no' and take him off every time he starts to hoist himself up. It's no good sometimes ignoring him and at other times getting mad. Take him off the table, state the rule 'You are not allowed to climb on the table' and find something else to distract him.

Toddler's memories are short and soon he will have forgotten about the table.

Consistency also means that you have the same rule for all places – in this case all tables – not just the dining table, but the coffee table in the lounge, the little one he does his drawings on in his room and any other table anywhere else at all. The same rule should apply to everyone else as well. Sally's mum has a rule about climbing on tables so when Sally's friend, Robert, starts to climb on the table Sally's mum lifts him off and says: 'You are not allowed to climb on the table.' It's the same rule for everyone.

Ask your friends and relatives to be consistent too. Ask them to back you up in your rule. It will not help you or your toddler if he is told by Mrs Williams next door that it's OK for him to sit on her patio table 'just this once'.

Which brings us neatly back to Rachel's problem at the beginning of this chapter. Rachel is sure what her rules are for Ben and Emily – no sweets before tea and no jumping on the bed – but she will need to be equally clear and consistent about her approach to her mother-in-law if her children are to feel comfortable staying with her. Toddlers prefer consistency.

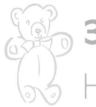

3
How to Head Off a Tantrum

If you see a tantrum on the horizon you may, just may, be able to head it off so long as you act quickly and decisively.

As we saw in Chapter 1, toddlers under about two and a half don't often give any warning of an impending tantrum, because frankly they don't know it's about to happen, but older toddlers are a little bit more self-aware, and often telegraph their intentions.

Distraction

Many parents try the old distraction standby of pointing off into the distance and saying 'Ooh look!' just when their toddler's face creases into the pre-tantrum 'But I want it my way' expression. It *can* work – but only for about a minute.

> The very first tantrum I can remember is nine-month-old Phoebe's "I'm not getting in my car seat" tizzy. At this age I thought it amusing that she could be bolshie! Usually a happy and contented little girl, she became a screaming, wriggling worm. Bribery worked at the time. I dangled car keys, tickled her and gave her a bottle to take her mind off the fact that I was strapping her in. Now that she's 11 months the process is no easier. Unless she's really tired she won't happily sit in her seat and, even though she's still small, no amount of wrestling and grappling will get her to bend in the middle and to sit to be strapped in. I am having to get cleverer at distracting her and she is becoming choosier at whether I will be successful or not.

Jo, mother of Phoebe, 11 months

You get slightly better results if you can jolly your toddler into some other involving activity. Once she is busy again she may just forget what she was worked up about.

> Jack always tantrums about holding my hand when out walking. Now I've bought some old-fashioned reins and we play racing horses to and from the shops!

Midge, mother of Jack, two

But sometimes, when you want her to do what you have asked her to do – eat tea or get out of the bath, for example – this sort of distraction isn't the answer.

If you want to make distraction work for you, you'll have to put your heart and soul into it. There are two techniques you can try:

- humour
- anger (fake it if you have to)

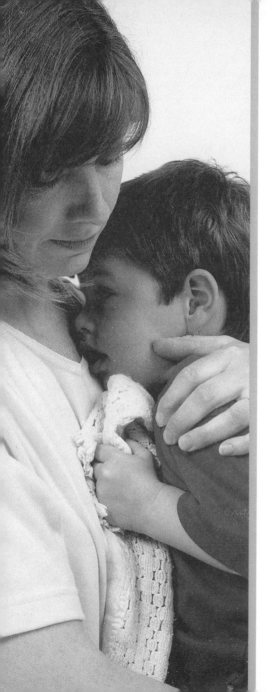

Humour

Toddlers love slapstick humour: grand gestures, funny voices and preposterous characters. For a distraction technique there's little to beat it. Humour works because:

- It makes your child laugh – and it's hard to be mean and moody when you're laughing.
- The sudden change from misery to laughter is such a surprise they are completely wrong-footed.
- Toddlers would rather laugh than cry, so there's no competition.
- It focuses your child on you, the clown, rather than on the problem.
- If you keep it up it can hook your child's imagination for long enough for her to forget what was bugging her before.
- It shows her how to make light of something she's struggling with – a good lesson for the future.
- It makes you feel good too.

Patrick (24 months) and Bethany (four) are sitting out the back having their tea. Bethany is tired and hungry after a busy day playing with new friends and is in no mood to tangle with Patrick who keeps snitching bits of bacon from her plate. Bethany starts to shout at Patrick who looks her straight in the eye and takes another piece. Bethany raises her arm to strike Patrick, but before things degenerate any further, Catherine, their mum, nips out the back door, a tea towel over her arm. 'Hey, signori, what is-a happening in this-a café?' She waves her arms about mock-Italian-style, and smiles broadly. 'There's-a shouting and a-screaming but not-a eating my beautiful food-a.' She claps her palm to her forehead and looks skyward; it's clear that she has missed her vocation and is thoroughly enjoying herself. 'Oh no-a, my beautiful food is still on the plates-a ...' and so on and on. Bethany and Patrick look at her open-mouthed (not a pretty sight) and finally laugh. They have no idea about restaurants or Italian waiters but they love the show, and now they are laughing, the squabbling is forgotten.

Sheila also finds that looking for the lighter side works:

> If I can make difficult situations into a game (which is usually quite hard work) then potential trouble spots can become good fun. For example Joseph has a little towelling bib with a picture of a monster on it. To get him to wear it, I tell him that a monster is going to eat up all the breakfast that drips down. He calls the bib the "muesli monster" now and that seems to relieve the stress of having to put it on.

Sheila, mother of Joseph, 20 months

The same technique works for Vicky on holiday with Simon (18 months) and Charlotte (three years old). But this time there's also a follow-through from the slapstick with a little bit of physical distraction to run off some of that excess energy that is just bursting to escape.

Charlotte is bored with the holiday routine of eating in the restaurant each night and has started to run around between courses. Vicky is embarrassed because none of the other children are doing this. But she also knows that insisting Charlotte keep her seat will trigger a tantrum. Charlotte already has a look of determination about her – a sure sign that the least little thing will set her off. Vicky leaves her seat and winks at Charlotte. 'Charlie,' she says, 'I'm going to sit out by the pool – want to come?' Charlotte is surprised because her mummy doesn't usually leave the table, but she goes happily.

Once outside, Vicky turns into a tour guide. 'Here we have the gorgeous pool, madam, for wearing your new bikini with the pink dots and very lovely you look too, if you don't mind my saying so.' Charlotte is staring at her mum and smiling. 'And here are the ever-so-comfy sun loungers ready for madam to lie down if she'd care to.' Charlotte lies down giggling. 'And oh, no! What's this? Two pesky mosquitoes have flown down and are dancing the tango on madam's tummy.' Vicky tickles Charlotte with both hands, and Charlotte screams and wriggles to be free, but the mosquitoes are insistent and tickle Charlotte all over until she is out of breath and helpless. Then Vicky and Charlotte sit and have a cuddle and talk about how boring restaurants can be, but how it's important not to spoil other people's meals and how next time they'll bring some things to play with. Then they go back in to their food.

The tickling has helped Charlotte to get rid of some surplus energy that would have made her tantrum a big one. Vicky feels good because she handled the situation well and she's had a laugh. (It's hard to tickle someone and not find it funny.)

But be warned – you need to pick your moment if you want to try physical distraction because tickling or even touching a toddler who is ready for a tantrum can sometimes hurl them straight into one. It's a little bit like a kind friend putting an arm around your shoulder when you are close to tears – it just makes you cry. It's usually safer to wait until your clowning has them rolling in the aisles before you move on to the audience participation bit.

Pillow fights and play fights can also work well. In fact, I still find these invaluable on long winter evenings, when it's too cold to go for a walk and tempers are running high. We pull the duvet down to the floor and gather armfuls of pillows from all the beds in the house and then we count one, two, three and all throw at once. After 10 minutes or so we only have energy enough to collapse on to the bed, still laughing, and cuddle. A great way to have fun. Alternatively, a good friend of mine pretends to pick up her toddler and empty all the cheekiness out of her toddler's head into the dustbin, and then yells into the dustbin 'Don't come back!' before slamming the lid down, dusting off her hands and smiling at her toddler.

Anger

I suppose this is the opposite of humour. Sort of an 'If they won't join you, beat them' approach. But humour and anger both work in the same way – to startle your toddler from her spiral down into a tantrum. But this time you beat her at her own game. You get in there first and you get angrier than she gets when her tantrum takes over.

Bob is bathing three-year-old Noel. They have had a great time with that old favourite of float-the-soap-on-the-rubber-duck-and-then-drop-the-flannel-from-a-great-height game. But now it is time to get out. Bob is holding up Noel's towel and Noel is having just one last go. The only trouble is that this is his fifth last go. Bob remembers last week when the same thing happened and he had to deal with tears and shouts and a lot of water going a lot of places he didn't want it to. He decides this time it's going to be different.

'OK that's it, out now,' he says, and Noel stops playing and looks at him, but it's only Dad and he doesn't have to worry so he goes back to his play. 'I said out now. How dare you not do what I say? I'm really angry now. Jump out of that bath immediately. I expect better from you. Now.' By this time Noel is scampering out of the bath as fast as he can. He didn't expect this. He can't match this. He'll do what he's told. Maybe once his dad stops yelling he can say sorry and they can be friends again. He hopes so. He likes the nice friendly Dad better. It was obviously really naughty to stay in the bath that long. He won't do that next time.

Of course, Bob gives Noel every opportunity to say sorry. Once Noel is bundled into his towel and being rubbed down Bob turns back into Mr Nice Guy again, so that as soon as Noel says sorry, Bob is able to say 'Thanks for that, Noel. I was really cross, but you got out quickly in the end. I know you'll be even quicker next time. We had a great play didn't we?' and off they go to brush Noel's teeth.

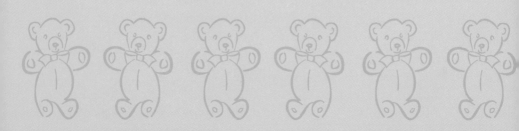

Bob has been angry, Noel has been shaken out of his tantrum, said sorry and now they are back to being friends again. It's all over and dealt with before it's begun. If you plan on using anger to motivate and surprise your toddler, make sure that you make friends with them soon after and that any apology they may offer is warmly accepted.

Don't teach them to sulk by holding against them the fact that you got angry.

Focusing on a Solution

There's very little point trying to reason with a toddler who's about to tantrum. Pre-tantrum toddlers have already lost most of their powers of reason, and trying to explain things or help sort things out will only make them feel less able to cope. This was the sort of mistake I made with my first child. I would spend ages reasoning with her – not able to see that she couldn't see what I was talking about. Finally I learnt from a younger but wiser friend to act decisively first and save the talking until she was on my wavelength again.

Once you have shouted or joked your toddler out of her would-be tantrum you should have her undivided attention for a few minutes. Some of the time you'll want to just get on with your day but at other times you'll feel that this is a good time to focus on the problem that nearly caused a tantrum. You can do this if you:

- Describe what happened ('You were about to hit your brother/You were running round the restaurant/You didn't get out of the bath when I asked you to …')
- Understand why it happened ('You didn't like Patrick taking your food/You were bored/You liked the game we were playing …')
- Say what you want to happen next time ('You choose some toys to bring to the table/You get out as soon as I ask you to …')

The older the toddler, the more of this information she can fill in for herself. Just ask:

- What happened back there?
- Why?
- What are you going to do next time?

You are getting your toddler to take responsibility for what she does. An essential skill for anyone who wants to be a real grown-up. For more on avoiding blame and excuses see Chapter 8.

When it's Better to Face a Tantrum

Naturally, with a toddler who tantrums frequently, you could spend a lot of time clowning or getting mad. But sometimes a tantrum may be just what the doctor ordered. If you feel you are treading on eggshells with your toddler you need to take steps to walk more firmly with her. If you're avoiding being firm because you just know she's going to explode then it is better to be firm. Stand firm and take the consequences. That way, at least you give yourself the chance to have some positively good times together, after the positively horrible ones are through. It's also important for your toddler that she does experience the full force of her own temper at least sometimes, so that she can see it won't destroy her.

There are two important and related principles involved in dealing with tantrums:

OK, not immediately – but given time. Toddlers are no exception. Toddlers need to be allowed to experience their failures so that they can move on. If your parenting is so seamless that your toddler never notices that the buckle she insisted on buckling stayed buckled not because she's a champion buckler but because you rebuckled it while she was struggling with her fleece, she'll miss out on five vital lessons:

- I can't do everything.
- Mum and Dad still love me even when I'm angry.

And eventually ...

- Not being able to do something is OK.
- I can cope with feeling I blew it.
- Nothing changes just because I want it to.

2 Making Things Better Doesn't Always Make Things Better

What toddlers need is the chance to work out a solution that suits them. If you always deflect a tantrum with another exciting adventure or a slapstick routine your toddler won't get the chance to draw on her own resources in finding a way around whichever dilemma she is currently facing. And finding alternative routes is one of the jobs of the toddler years. This is why it's sometimes OK to let your toddler cry and scream – because tears and shouts are an expression of sadness and frustration that are often quickly followed by new solutions.

The truth is that you can't make everything better for your toddler and you shouldn't try either.

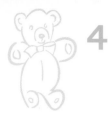

4

Tantrum Hotspots

You can recognize the triggers that are likely to lead to tantrums. Tantrums can happen anyplace, anytime, but they are much more likely when:

- You can't give your toddler your undivided attention.
- Your toddler is feeling stressed through hunger, illness, tiredness, boredom or simply the demands of being little.

Baby Blues

Many toddlers revert to more infantile behaviour and tantrum more when their parents have a new baby. Toddlers do this because your new baby is creaming off some of the attention that used to be theirs and they figure:

- 'That baby is getting what should be mine. How can I get the attention back? I know, act like a baby …'
- 'I can't manage on my own. I'll have to show Mum and Dad what it feels like to be me …'

But even though you understand it, this sort of babyish behaviour can be frustrating. Particular trouble spots include:

- Reverting to wet pants and puddles when he has been dry for months
- Waking at night when he has slept right through for ages (especially when you've just settled the baby in his cot for the fifth time)
- Preferring to use fingers when eating or to have you feed him.

Other toddlers respond to a baby brother or sister by stealing a biscuit here or a yoghurt there. Some experts believe this is a toddler's way of looking for the love he feels he has lost to his younger sibling. But it's no good you asking him why he is stealing – he doesn't know.

Toddlers with smaller siblings often have to wait for things they want – a play with mum, a cuddle, or their tea – especially when there is only one parent around. Sometimes your toddler can do things on his own while you are busy, and sometimes you can include him in the things that you are doing – he can 'read' his book to you while you feed the baby, or change his dolly while you change his brother. At other times he can be a helper – bringing you the baby's bib or playing with the baby while you pick up the toys. But although learning to share and to wait are valuable lessons for your toddler, it's important for him that now and again you stop juggling his needs and just be with him.

From time to time the baby can wait. A crying baby is telling you that he needs something, but your toddler has needs too. Your toddler needs to know that sometimes he comes first. One good way to make sure he knows is to play with him even when the baby cries but to ask *him* to tell *you* when he thinks you ought to feed the baby. (If the baby cries loudly enough he'll want you to feed him pretty soon.)

Unfortunately, there's no immediate fix for these problems. We all take time to adjust to a new human being in our lives. Probably the best advice is to treat your toddler like a baby again, when he wants to be. Nobody likes to feel that they have to be capable and in control the whole time – it's just too much of a burden. But there need to be limits to what you will accept. The best thing you can do is to be firm about your rules:

- 'I expect you to tell me when you need a wee.'
- 'Here is your bed. Go to sleep now. I'll see you in the morning.'
- 'You get more jelly in your tummy if you use the spoon, rather than your fingers.'

The clearer you can be, the safer he will feel. And ensure you have lots of fun times just with the two of you, when he can be just how he wants – a little baby or a big boy. Let him know by the amount and the quality of time you spend together, as well as telling him directly, that you still love him just as much as you did, and that he is still just as special to you.

Tantrums Outside the House

Enter any supermarket on a sunny afternoon and you're likely to hear at least one toddler in full tantrum, and another two or three gearing up in readiness. Supermarkets have all the necessary ingredients for command performance tantrums. There you are, *with* him and yet busy, probably distracted and everything takes a lot longer than you thought (especially as you inevitably forget to pick up the baked beans on aisle 3 and only remember them when you hit the bread on aisle 18).

He starts off wanting to help – squeezing the tomatoes to check they are ripe, selecting you the best tin of beans, running his fingers along the bottles of wine, pleading with you to go back to look at that picture of Thomas the Tank Engine on the cereal packet. But once past the sweetie aisle, his enthusiasm quickly wanes and you're torn. Either you can race round at top speed ignoring him and risking a tantrum, or slow down so that he feels involved, making you late for everything else.

Here are six ways to avoid supermarket tantrums:

- Top tip:

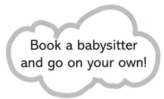

Book a babysitter and go on your own!

- Swop toddlers with a friend and go to different supermarkets – your cherub is less likely to play her up, and you'll be surprised how angelic your friend's toddler can be.
- Try starting with short trips and build up to long hauls gradually. Let him practise doing without your undivided attention.
- Take him a selection of books, cuddly toys and nutritious snacks to divert him.
- Talk about all the purchases you're making – if he's already two years old let him help you find the orange juice, cereal, pizzas. Just make sure you're standing pretty close at first as long searches will frustrate him.
- Let him choose within limits – 'Shall we get red apples or green apples this week?' 'Do you prefer the white or the pink toilet paper?' This is more time-consuming, but it keeps the two of you talking (which is what your toddler likes).

But if, in spite of all this, your toddler throws a wobbly, what can you do?

Toddlers love an audience, and supermarkets are one enormous stage. But it's not just our toddlers who play to the gallery. As parents we feel on show too and this affects the way that we behave, both before a tantrum begins and when one is in full swing.

> We were at the supermarket in Hammersmith – my husband, my stepdaughter, Lynne, and her boyfriend and we were pushing Jamie around on the trolley and he started yelling, I don't know what for he just did. He yelled and yelled and I tried to calm him down, but he just carried on. Well, I hate toddlers crying, but I wasn't embarrassed. After a minute I turned round to talk to Lynne but all three adults had sneaked out of the shop and were hiding outside, with embarrassment!

Sue, mother of Jamie, two

Naturally, our toddlers, being the bright, perceptive characters we always hoped they'd be, sense that we feel uneasy being watched and act accordingly.

There are four reasons why handling tantrums outside the home is tougher than within our four walls:

- There's always at least one person watching your every move.
- You may feel embarrassed and helpless as well as angry.
- The most effective option of walking away from your toddler isn't possible.
- You know that you are partly responsible for the tantrum (you brought them into the supermarket, didn't you?) so you don't feel quite as decisive.

Sarah, mother of Harriet (aged three), says that she feels quite different when Harriet throws a tantrum in the supermarket:

> At home I feel "Oh, God not again", but at least I can just walk away calmly – well, fairly calmly. But when we're out it's just so embarrassing and even though people don't usually say anything I can feel their eyes boring into the back of my head. I can hear myself saying things louder than I need to just for their benefit. I still walk away and stand waiting for her to finish just round the corner from where she is but it's definitely much worse when we're out.

Sarah, mother of Harriet, three

In many ways, Sarah is doing the best she can in difficult circumstances. An audience always changes a performance. Have the courage of your convictions – you know what you need to do. (There is some good advice on this in Chapter 5.) The same things that work at home will work when you're out. Hang on to that knowledge and don't change your script to suit your critics.

> Last week we were out shopping, queuing up to pay. Rebecca wanted to be in the toy shop which we'd been bribing her with all the way round the shops. Finally, she decided she'd had enough, lay on her back on the floor, kicked her legs, and cried and shouted. So, as the queue moved forward I stepped over her and went ahead with the queue to pay, leaving her lying on the floor. My mother, who was with me, was amazed at how calm I was. Everyone else ignored her as well. I paid and then gathered her up into the buggy and off we went and she was OK. I think this was the first time I've done it right. Before now I've gathered her up immediately and tried to pacify her but then the thing would just escalate and she'd cry more. It's definitely better to let the paddy have its run.

Lindsey, mother of Rebecca, two

Sometimes you can even use some of that frustration you feel to fuel an answer to nosey passers-by, as Alice did:

> Tom threw a real wobbly in a shop because I wouldn't buy the biggest box of crayons. He was screaming and kicking when a grandmotherly voice behind me said "Poor boy. He wants the crayons and he can't have them." I was so cross someone was interfering that I spun round and said "No he can't and it's my job as his mother to make sure he doesn't learn that having a tantrum is the way to get what he wants!" I felt much better that everyone looking knew that I was doing something positive.

Alice, mother of Tom, 18 months

Talking on the Phone

It's one of the laws of parenthood that your toddler will need you most urgently as soon as you answer the phone. Wherever he was when the phone rang, and whatever he was doing, he will suddenly find that you are the one person in the world he needs, and now. Personally, I am eternally grateful to the inventor of the portable phone. I have lost track of the number of times I have changed a nappy, wiped a bottom, found a biscuit or retrieved some essential toy from under the washing machine while talking on the phone.

You can't avoid phone calls altogether. If you tried, you'd leave yourself isolated and unhappy. However, there are ways you can minimize their tantrum potential:

- Keep them short.
- Agree to call the other person back in two minutes (or ask them to call you) and in the meantime find something absorbing for your toddler to do.
- Be clear that this isn't his time. Say 'Excuse me a minute' to your caller and then give your full attention to your toddler as you tell him that although you would love to talk about the cat/look at the spider in the kitchen/find his hat with the pink flowers you are in fact on the phone. Give him some suggestions about what he can do, a time limit for yourself for the call and the hope that you will be there for him soon.

Now You See Me, Now You Don't

Saying 'Hello' and 'Goodbye' can cause tantrums too. Which is why many tantrums happen at the beginning and end of events. Tantrums often flare up at the beginning or end of:

- playgroup
- visits to friends/the park/anything else enjoyable
- bedtime
- bathtime
- dressing/undressing

In fact, stopping or starting any activity at all may result in a tantrum. Some toddlers (and a lot of bigger people too) rush to begin things, and are always more than ready to end, whereas others are extremely anxious to begin with and then, having begun, find it hard to stop. Those in the second group are more likely to have tantrums at the end of one activity and at the start of another. Louise knows which group Matty is in:

'Matty loves her swimming lesson, especially the last half-hour when all the toys come out. On this particular occasion, she wouldn't get out of the pool. I had to drag her out, screaming, and she continued to scream all through the showers and the changing room! She was thrashing about on the floor of the changing room with all the other mothers politely trying to ignore us! I had to hold her down forcibly to get her nappy on, and found I'd left awful red marks on her lily-white skin. She then jumped up and ran, semi-naked, screaming and covered with red marks, out of the changing rooms, through the leisure centre and down to the cafeteria, where she gave up.'

Louise, mother of Matty, 33 months

One way to head off a tantrum is to give your toddler a five-minute warning. This is especially important for toddlers who don't like change. Let him know that what he is doing now has to end soon and, if you can, spend the next five minutes with him bringing everything to a close. You won't have to do this forever, just until he learns to take care of the endings for himself.

If he's having a bath and often screams when you need to jump him out, help him spend five minutes beforehand putting his toys back in their places for the night and watching the water swirl around the plughole. Sometimes singing a song about the disappearing water helps, or telling him the story of the water once it leaves the bath. Turn jumping out into a game by whizzing him out like a rocket, or jumping him like a kangaroo, and as you do so, talk to him about the nice things to come – a warm towel, an en-OR-mous cuddle, some clean pyjamas or whatever.

'I used to dread bathtimes. Luke would stay in for an hour and still tantrum when it was time to come out. One evening I got an old fluffy brown towel from the airing cupboard and suggested he might like to be a big brown bear. Luke hopped straight out and growled happily while I dried him!'

Deidre, mother of Luke, 26 months

You may find that spending the first five minutes, as well as the last five, of any activity with your toddler gives him the confidence to feel that moving on is OK, and that ultimately he can manage this on his own and enjoy it. So, if your toddler often tantrums at bedtime, reassure him that you will spend an extra five minutes with him just talking about his teddies, or the picture on his duvet, the patterns he can see when he closes his eyes, the dreams he might dream or anything else connected with the business of getting ready to sleep.

One of the biggest changes that some toddlers have to deal with is coping when you leave them in someone else's care. Picture the scene: you arrive at your regular childminder's home. Your toddler gives you a hug and toddles off into the back room, you call out 'Bye, sweetheart, see you later. Have a good time.' But before you can hand over the nappy-changing bag, spare clothes, teddy and tell his minder what time you'll be picking him up, he's back, clinging to your leg and talking in his small voice – a sure sign that with very little provocation he'll collapse into a tantrum. Sounds familiar? You're not alone. But what should you do?

Firstly, don't be governed by guilt. Guilt trips often stop us acting in ways that are reasonable and fair. There isn't a working parent who hasn't felt guilty at some point about leaving their child to go to work. But your guilt alone doesn't mean that you shouldn't work. If there's no good reason for you not to go, then go. Have a brief, warm hug, say goodbye and leave – just as you would have done if your toddler had been happy to see you go. The tantrum, if there is one, will have stopped before you've turned the first corner. It was for your benefit, and without the audience there's not a lot of mileage in an extended performance.

If you don't feel happy with the childminder or your toddler is ill, those are separate matters, and you must deal with them. Don't wait for him to tantrum before you do what you know you should have done all along.

Playgroups and nurseries are a similar large break from your care for your older toddler. Childminders and nursery school teachers see more toddlers tantrum at setting-down and at picking-up times than at any other times during the session. This fits in with what we know about tantrums – that they are to do with the relationship between you and your toddler. Once you've gone, most toddlers have no reason to tantrum. However, there are a few toddlers who do tantrum when their parents aren't about. Playgroup leaders say that these toddlers usually come from families that are feeling the stress of:

- illness
- marital tension
- the birth of a sibling
- moving house
- a death in the family
- financial worries

The more of these stresses you have to cope with, the harder it is. The sad truth is that stress can fracture families. Stress can pull you in every direction except closer. When everyone is stressed, it can be hard for your toddler to find a special place for himself in the family and this feeling of drifting makes tantrums more likely.

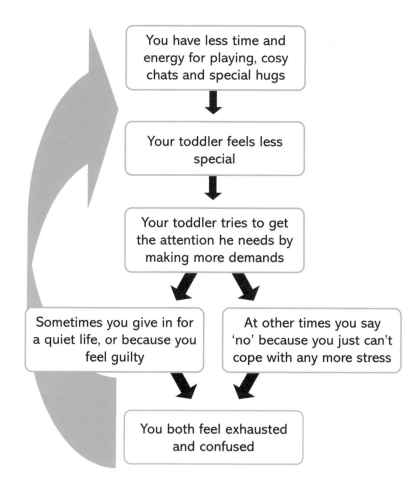

You have less time and energy for playing, cosy chats and special hugs

↓

Your toddler feels less special

↓

Your toddler tries to get the attention he needs by making more demands

Sometimes you give in for a quiet life, or because you feel guilty

At other times you say 'no' because you just can't cope with any more stress

You both feel exhausted and confused

Tantrums at nursery may be your toddler's way of showing you that he doesn't feel he's getting the firm, fair, loving care he needs from you. They may be his way of asking the firm, fair and loving adults at nursery to help him out, to give him what you can't manage right now. These sort of tantrums are a clear message that you need to act.

You could:

- spend more time with him having fun and being close – let him take the lead for half an hour or so
- give him more hugs and kisses and remind him often that you love him
- focus on him as an individual
- be consistent
- listen to his demands – if they are reasonable go with them; if they are unreasonable refuse

If you are unsure what is reasonable and what is not, see Chapter 2.

Special Needs

In nurseries that cater for children with special needs, tantrums within the sessions are more common. The reasons for this are that:

- It's harder for parents of children with special needs to decide on appropriate limits to behaviour, and harder to stick to them.
- Life is more frustrating for children with special needs either because they can't express themselves, can't physically do what they would like to, or can't understand why they have to do certain things.
- Children with developmental delay behave in ways which are a couple of years or more younger than their chronological age.

When life is difficult it's even more important to be consistent in your approach. That way, at least you and your toddler can rely on some things always being the same. It will take much longer for your toddler with special needs to understand what he can and cannot do and what he can and cannot have but you will only make it harder for him by giving in now and again. But be kind to yourself. Take support and encouragement from the staff at the nursery and make sure you have some time to yourself each day. Your toddler needs you well and happy.

Getting Dressed

Some toddlers love the challenge of getting dressed and others are happy to stand still while you do it for them. Others still, fight you every inch of the way – not wanting you to do it and refusing to do it themselves.

It can be a fraught business. If you are doing it:

- make it fun
- sing a getting-dressed song as you go
- make a game of it. You could say 'Oh, where are those hands/feet/head?' as they disappear through sleeves/trousers/tops and 'Oh, there they are' as they reappear

If she wants to choose her clothes:

- Put away all those completely impossible items – the sundress with the crossover straps where she always pokes her head through the sleeve hole or the much-loved, but way too small and frankly past it, T-shirt from holiday.
- Limit her choice and then respect her decision.
- Leave more time than you think it could possibly take (successful management consultants always plan a job and then triple their original estimate of the time).

It's always difficult to get things right for a toddler, even, as Isaac's mum Jane says, when you do something that's worked before:

The other day I put out suitable clothes for going to nursery on a warm day – ones that on other days there'd been no problem with. But this day Isaac put his trousers and pants on and then said that they felt funny and began thrashing his legs. Well, I just said "Put your clothes on. There is nothing wrong with them, they are perfectly all right. Stop screaming." This got results, in the sense that he got dressed, but he still screamed for another 10 minutes.

Sometimes at the weekend, when the same thing happens, I say "OK, you choose" and then he is much quicker to calm down. But the stupid thing is that sometimes he will choose the same clothes that the previous day had made him throw a wobbly! I have to admit that letting him choose is definitely easier – but it depends on my mood. Sometimes I just want to win – that's how I feel – so I do persist in a confrontation. Sometimes I want to stamp my authority, in preparation for later life.

Jane, mother of Isaac, four and a half

Jim has a similar problem with Jack:

Every morning Jack wants to put on his favourite tracksuit of the moment and gets upset when it's in the laundry. Sometimes he even hunts through the dirty washing, and tells us he got the clothes from the ironing pile. He gets so obsessive that in the past Grace has even hidden some of his clothes once they were washed, so that he can't find them. Then we have a great set-to over that as well. Tears and shouting – and that's just us. At night there is often a fight to get him into the bath, not because he doesn't like to be clean, but more because he knows his clothes will disappear into the laundry basket. But he's taken a leaf out of our book and sometimes hides his clothes from us so that we can't get them.

Jim, father of Jack, four

When life gets to be a series of battles it may be worth sitting down with your toddler and explaining things simply, or working out a compromise.

If he wants to dress himself:

- Initially, at least, stay with him while he gets dressed. That way, if those pants do get themselves in a twist, you'll be ready to lend a hand.
- So long as he's happy, stand back — no matter how clumsy he seems.
- Don't laugh.
- Don't criticize.
- It's my firm belief that socks were invented by people who like tormenting toddlers, so be ready to whip those awkward beasties over your toddler's heels once he has pulled them over his toes.

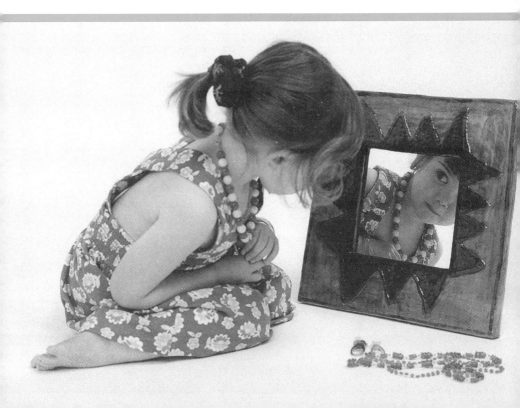

If he's dilly-dallying deliberately and time has run out:

- Lift him and carry him and his remaining clothes to the front door. Get him dressed there, where 'going out' will be the obvious next step.
- If he refuses to wear a coat, let him experience that chill winds make him cold.

If you have a bad time at the supermarket/playgroup/childminder's one day, you may feel anxious about going again. Your toddler may too. Toddlers, just like us, learn from experience and use what they have learnt to predict the future. Try to work out which part of the experience made him tantrum before a pattern develops:

- If he was bored, maybe you could take more toys.
- If he was hungry, provide little snacks.
- If he finds it hard to say goodbye, give him advance warning that you will be going in two minutes and make sure he has already made contact with another adult before you say goodbye.

Kitty's mum Dawn has her own solution:

We used to have the classic supermarket checkout tantrum when I wouldn't let Kitty have the sweets she wanted. Now I always buy a packet of mini-doughnuts on the way in and give her one or two as we go round.

Dawn, mother of Kitty, two and a half

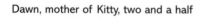

Food

Food can trigger toddler tantrums in two ways. Hunger and food refusal. Let's take them in that order.

Hunger

The toddler-food motto is 'little and often'. Toddlers need regular snacks between meals to keep them happy and busy. Carry snacks with you on days out, or when collecting him from a morning activity. Fruit, sandwiches and lumps of cheese are almost as easy as crisps, biscuits and sweets and a lot better nutritionally. Food offered in this way, as though it were a treat, is often eaten more readily than food presented after hours spent in the kitchen. Which brings me on to the other food issue for toddlers.

Food Refusal

Toddlers love to say 'no'. It helps them feel in control. Food is a great boon for your toddler because he learns pretty quickly that there is no way you can force him to eat, so he can say 'no' and win. Over and above outright refusal, toddlers often develop rituals about what and in which way they will eat. All toddlers have, at some point, refused to eat one of the following:

- meat, because it is touching the vegetables
- pasta, because the sauce is poured on top
- a yoghurt that he did not open herself
- sandwiches that are cut in squares and not triangles
- any food at all unless it is on a Winnie-the-Pooh plate
- the same food as yesterday
- different food from yesterday ...

... and on and on and on. It's so easy to get things wrong with a toddler at mealtimes that it's probably best to go along with his whims and fancies most of the way, and only hold out for the absolute essentials. If you know that he doesn't like yoghurt with bits in don't give him yoghurt with bits in for now, just thank your lucky stars he eats yoghurt at all. If you know it matters to him which chair he sits in – ask first. If you can try to meet his requests most of the time for a while, he may be prepared to accept it when you can't.

Sonia has her own method for encouraging Patrick to eat. 'If he makes a fuss about finishing his dinner I just give him his pudding too and he eats everything at the same time.'

Be firm about the behaviours that really matter to you; things like throwing or spitting food, running around while eating or upending drinks. Be prepared to weather the tantrums that erupt when you insist on these social conventions.

Remember, a normal toddler will not starve herself, and that all foods, even crisps, biscuits and bowls of cereal, contain some nutrition. But if you are worried about the range and the quality of food your toddler eats, your health visitor is a good person to talk to.

When your child has finished eating, no matter how soon that is, remove his plate and let him get down to play. Making him sit at table with nothing to do will make him bored and is asking for trouble.

Tiredness and Boredom

Two minutes can be a long time for a toddler if they don't have something engrossing to do. Having to wait even a short time can lead to a tantrum. Reduce tiredness and boredom by:

- Breaking up his activities into short chunks. (The average two-year-old can concentrate for 12 minutes at a time.)
- Increasing his attention span by playing alongside him or chatting to him as he plays.
- Not expecting too much of your toddler.
- Stopping to look at interesting things when you are out for a walk.
- Keeping the horizon close on walks, especially on the way back – once a tired toddler sees that the end is a long way off he feels twice as tired! Keep to walks with lots of corners. Anne does this by building in familiar landmarks: 'On a long walk home we have regular stopping spots so I can say "Let's run to the street name post" or "Will we see the squirrel in the tree?" or "When we get to the crossing, you can push the button."'
- Making sure he has time to potter. If he has had a busy morning at the park, at a friend's house or just at the supermarket, he needs a quiet afternoon at home with you. Pottering is an essential part of your toddler's day.

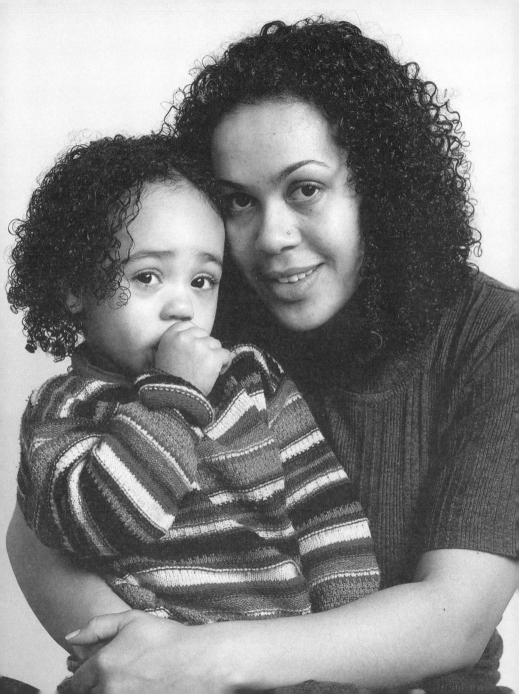

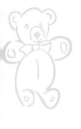

5
How to Handle a Tantrum

Get this right and your toddler will have fewer tantrums and be more able to deal with her emotional highs and lows in a reasonable way.

Treat her as though you know she will be able to pass through this stage, and she will come through confident and sure that you understand her. Give her the impression that you can't cope with her displays of frustration and anger and she will feel that everything is out of control. Toddlers who feel this way go on repeating the pattern of emotional extremes, hoping that someone, somewhere will be able to contain them.

Of course, the best way to manage a tantrum is to remain adult, caring, positive and consistent throughout. But it's never an easy task and it gets harder the older your toddler is. With young toddlers the tantrum is often so quick and so immediately and easily forgotten that it's difficult to see what all the fuss is about, but older toddlers have more sticking power and have learnt how to fine-tune their tantrums to ensure maximum effect. If you blow it one day try not to beat yourself up about it. Remember, you'll probably have a lot more opportunities to get it right!

Setting Limits

Your toddler needs you to limit her behaviour. If you don't tell her clearly and firmly what is and isn't on she'll go on pushing every time you say 'no' to find out if you mean it this time. It's easier to set limits as soon as the first tantrum occurs than to wait until she's a tyrannical three-and-a-half-year-old. Get in first, get in early and your life will be your own. Give in 'just this once' and your toddler will hope that every time will be 'just this once'. Make up your mind now – there's no such thing as 'just this once'. It isn't naughtiness that makes her yell and scream to get what she wants – it's you. Inconsistency leads to more and worse tantrums which can go on for years.

Calm and clear limits are the best sort. If you're yelling 'How many times do I have to tell you …?' maybe you didn't say it calmly and clearly in the first place.

Of course, most of us get to this stage at times. When you do it can help if you:

- Count to 10 before you say anything else.
- Shout out how you feel, rather than what you want your toddler to do.
- Walk away and get rid of that fury somewhere safer – try thumping a pillow or a teddy.

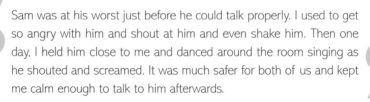

Sam was at his worst just before he could talk properly. I used to get so angry with him and shout at him and even shake him. Then one day, I held him close to me and danced around the room singing as he shouted and screamed. It was much safer for both of us and kept me calm enough to talk to him afterwards.

Rose, mother of Sam, two

Whatever her age your toddler needs to feel that you are in control of yourself and of her. She needs to feel 'held' by the way that you deal with her anger and frustration, so that eventually she can hold herself together enough to come back alongside you. If you do blow your top and end up having your own tantrum, show her that you can recover and be kind to yourself by apologizing to her and then doing something together that you both enjoy.

Your toddler needs to feel that you love her, but you don't like the tantrum.

There are three steps to making this clear:

- stand firm
- 'time out' – either walk away or hold tight (see page 73)
- afterwards – a hug, with or without a punishment, but always a hug

Standing Firm

If you take only one piece of advice from this book take this – don't give in to a tantrum – ever. You are the boss, you have a right to have your toddler fit in with your requests. You know more than she does and you have her best interests at heart. Whereas she only wants what she wants.

Of course, she has a right to expect you to be reasonable. If you say 'no' to everything she wants without giving it a second thought, you can expect more tantrums. It's hard for any of us to cope when those we love don't listen to even our reasonable requests.

Standing firm means saying 'no' and staying calm. If you yell or shout to get your point across you may scare your toddler but she won't know what you are yelling about. This is the time to become the strong, silent type.

Most of us have said 'no' and then wished we'd said 'yes' at some time or other. If you decide you were wrong to say 'no' but the tantrum has already started don't give in – insist that she accepts your decision. Saying 'yes' now will only convince her that the tantrum changed your mind. Hold out for what you originally said. But next time make sure you think beforehand. Does it really matter if she has five minutes longer at her friend's house, removes all the pans from the cupboard, wears odd socks or is it just you that can't cope with handing over this much control?

If you get it wrong, let the tantrum run its course and then apologize. We all make mistakes, but it's important that we say sorry, so that we and our children can learn from it. An apology is one of the greatest bonds between a toddler and a parent. When our children see that we are fallible, and admit it, they love us more. Eventually they learn to accept their own mistakes too.

Time Out

Tantrums are your toddler's way of expressing how she feels when she can't get your attention. To teach her that this isn't an acceptable way to catch your eye you need to make sure that you don't give her any attention while the tantrum is in full throttle. The best way to do this is with time out. Time out means that you withhold your attention until she is ready to be reasonable again. It's up to you whether you hold her tight (see page 73) until she's all played out or walk away.

Separating Yourself

Lots of parents walk away from their toddler when she throws a tantrum. It works. But it works best when you do it calmly, and ignore even the 'best' advice to the contrary:

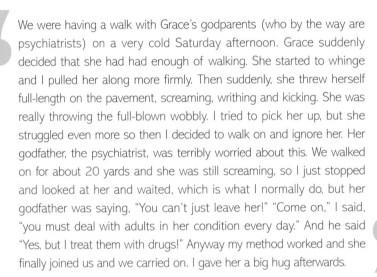

We were having a walk with Grace's godparents (who by the way are psychiatrists) on a very cold Saturday afternoon. Grace suddenly decided that she had had enough of walking. She started to whinge and I pulled her along more firmly. Then suddenly, she threw herself full-length on the pavement, screaming, writhing and kicking. She was really throwing the full-blown wobbly. I tried to pick her up, but she struggled even more so then I decided to walk on and ignore her. Her godfather, the psychiatrist, was terribly worried about this. We walked on for about 20 yards and she was still screaming, so I just stopped and looked at her and waited, which is what I normally do, but her godfather was saying, "You can't just leave her!" "Come on," I said, "you must deal with adults in her condition every day." And he said "Yes, but I treat them with drugs!" Anyway my method worked and she finally joined us and we carried on. I gave her a big hug afterwards.

Shirley, mother of Grace, 33 months

If your toddler is lying on the floor screaming and drumming her heels, make sure she is safe where she is and then simply step over her and do something else. Try to do this as quietly as you can. Make as little fuss as possible. The less attention you give her the better. If you look or glare at her, or talk or more probably yell at her to be quiet, to be reasonable or to just hold on, she has got what she wants – your attention. It may convince her that the tantrum is worth it. Even if you yell 'Right, that's it' as you slam the door and leave, you have still attended to her tantrum. It's far better to pretend that nothing is happening and completely ignore her. Let the tantrum run its course and then deal with the aftermath.

Debbie, an experienced nursery teacher, who runs a special-needs nursery, does just this. When children tantrum during a session, she carries on with the other children as though the tantrumming child doesn't exist. When the screaming is dying down she goes over to the toddler, bends down and says 'When you are ready to join in again, we're right here.' Then she turns away again, but stays close. Within a minute most toddlers are back in the group and smiling. Neat work.

Dawn did the same when Kitty refused to walk home from the shops:

> We used to fight about walking home from the supermarket. Kitty would just stand still. I'd be loaded with shopping and her brother would be running ahead. I had it out with her one day. I sat on a nearby wall for over 20 minutes. It was more a battle of wills than a tantrum and I won. Since then there haven't been any more problems – at least not about walking home.

Dawn, mother of Kitty, three and a half

It's important not to keep returning to the scene of the crime. Don't keep checking to see if she's coming out of it – the performance will just last longer. Do something that might under other circumstances (were it not for the wailing that is going on nearby) absorb or relax you – put the headphones on and listen to some music, make yourself a coffee or read the paper – it may work so long as you can shut out some of the noise. Alternatively, get rid of some of that pent-up energy and anger you are feeling by dancing vigorously, thumping your sofa cushions or running up and down stairs as fast as you can – preferably out of sight of your toddler, or she will see that she has hooked you into her tantrum.

Holding Tight

Other parents prefer to hold their toddler tightly during a tantrum, and again it works. In fact, when you're out, often it's the only alternative. But if you are going for the holding technique you have to feel in control of your own emotions. Only hold your toddler if you feel you can do so without injuring her. Holding your toddler should make her feel secure, not powerless. If you can only do it through clenched teeth don't do it at all. Of course, she will struggle to be free of you, and you must be ready to defend yourself from the thrashing of her limbs, but in the end when her tantrum is all gone she and you will be well placed for a hug. Your aim is to hold her tight – squeeze the tantrum out quickly, rather than allowing it to linger. Be a still centre to her storm. A safe haven to which she can finally return.

> Holding didn't work with my first child: he was just too violent, but it did work with Katy. She didn't tantrum often, but when she did it was a monster one and she ended up sobbing and shaking. I would hold her firmly throughout and during the shaky phase – it was just what she needed. She would even fall asleep in my arms sometimes.
>
> **Emily, mother of Katy, two**

If you go for holding you have a choice about the way you do it:

- emotional absence
- emotional connection

Emotional Absence

If you need to cut yourself off from the screams and punches of your toddler in order to get through the tantrum, that's fine. While you are holding her either look away or stare coolly at her. Be there for her physically, but absent in spirit. Do not smile or stroke; do not comfort or cajole. This is all attention and your toddler will feel she has gained by her tantrum. She fell into this tantrum because she couldn't cope with not being able to have all of you – mind and body, so don't give it to her now, or she will feel that a tantrum is a reasonable way to get her needs met. Stare at her blankly or not at all and she will quickly see that tantrums get her nothing that she wants.

Emotional Connection

But if the effort of pretending that you're not concerned leaves you boiling inside it's better to talk about feelings throughout the tantrum. Much of parenting is learning how to take care of ourselves so that we can be there for our children. Talking through a tantrum allows you to hold yourself as well as your toddler, not just with your arms but with your voice and your thoughts too. In fact, if physically holding your toddler seems too dangerous (and many toddlers are very violent when in a tantrum) sitting close by but holding your toddler in your heart and mind may be the safest option.

Take Gina. Gina is 22 months old, vivacious, creative and wilful. She has just decided to use her paints in the lounge and her mum, Sarah, has asked her to move them to the kitchen, where the floor is washable. Gina refuses. Mum offers the kitchen or the backyard. Gina refuses, and Mum takes the paints into the kitchen. Gina throws herself to the floor and screams; her legs kick away the remaining pieces of paper and the jar of brushes. Sarah is exasperated. Painting wasn't part of her plan anyway so even painting in the kitchen is a concession. She feels like throwing the paints, paper and brushes in the bin and banishing Gina to her room for the rest of the day. She controls the impulse and, after watching Gina yell for a few more seconds, she kneels on the floor and says quietly to Gina: 'Boy, I am so cross with you, I feel I'm going to explode.'

Gina, of course, can't hear her because she's screaming so loudly. But Sarah knows that. This talking, this emotional picture that Sarah is painting of the tantrum and the feelings that lie behind it is for her, not for Gina. It will allow her to be ready to meet Gina's needs once Gina finally stops yelling. This is why she talks quietly, rather than trying to beat Gina at her own game by shouting. Shouting at your toddler during a tantrum is a waste of time – she can't hear you and you may just scare her more. 'I am really mad, and so are you. We're two angry people. And you have no idea how much I wish I could lie down on the floor and just let it all hang out like you.'

Sarah stops, she has accepted how she feels and how Gina feels and has said what the little girl inside her would like to be able to do. She looks at Gina with her red face and her open mouth, tears streaming down her cheeks and she says quietly: 'You are cross with me because you had a great idea and I said "no" ... You wanted to paint in the lounge where it is sunny and I said you had to go to the dark kitchen ... I squashed your idea and now you feel squashed too ...'

Sarah sits and looks at Gina, who is calming down a little. She also feels a little calmer. Sarah feels she understands a little bit better what Gina might be going through now. 'It's very hard to be a mum when you have to say "no" to something good like painting. And it's hard to be a very little girl who has to do what her mum says. We'll get there in the end, we'll get there.' Sarah sits in silence. She has acknowledged how hard all this is, for both of them. She has accepted Gina's frustration and her own and is ready to hug Gina when Gina finally crawls over to her.

Sarah's monologue helps her to make sense of her own feelings and Gina's feelings. It also helps her keep in touch with what is really going on for both of them. Although Gina will not be able to hear what is being said, the fact that Sarah has sat with her throughout will have had an impact. She will have felt held. At some level she will know that Sarah is there, holding her while she cannot hold herself, ready to welcome her back.

Every time your toddler is frustrated, expresses it in a tantrum, and survives, she grows a little more realistic, a little more certain of her ability to withstand violent emotions and a little more certain of your ability to love her in spite of her bawling 'I hate you' at the top of her voice. Toddlers need to know that you love them enough to listen to them as they experience hateful emotions. They also need to know that you are big enough to take it without collapsing or yelling back. This way your toddler can gradually learn to accept it too.

Nicky found that this approach worked with Patrick:

Not long after his little sister was born Patrick (two and a half) had a tantrum on the upstairs landing, but I really can't remember what triggered it off. He was beating his fists, drumming his heels and shouting "No!" It was a classic. It was late afternoon, a bad time for all of us. He got himself into such a state that he was frightening himself. I said "Can you tell me what you're cross about?" I think it helps to name the emotions for a two-year-old just as you would name the colours and the numbers. It's about the only tantrum he's had so far.

Nicky, mother of Patrick, two and a half

- Accept and say how you feel. For example: 'I feel furious/helpless/exhausted.'
- Watch your toddler. Describe how she seems. For example: 'You look fragile/desperate. You sound tired/angry.'
- Show you understand how tough it is for her. For example: 'It must be hard not being able to explain what you want/Maybe it feels as though I say "no" to everything you think of/Maybe you just need to show me you're not ready to be grown up all the time yet.'
- Express your confidence in yourself and your toddler. For example: 'I know that we'll sort this one out.'

One of the spin-offs of keeping in touch with your feelings is that less often you feel like forcing the issue and smacking your toddler into submission. Physical blows destroy a child's already fragile sense of herself, so that she shrinks away from all the other love and care you have to offer. As a caring parent your aim is to help and guide her to become a loving, open, warm and authoritative adult – in fact just like you are, most of the time. She can't learn to be like the warm and kind you if she's busy hiding from your smacks. And just in case you're not convinced, there is researched hard evidence to show that toddlers who are hit for a tantrum not only have more tantrums, but become either bullies or victims. Smacking not only doesn't work, it makes toddlers worse.

Deciding to give up smacking is a brave idea. Actually giving it up is a harder task. When smacking is a habit it's often difficult to see what else you could do instead. Smacking is often something that we learn from our parents – they smacked us so we smack our children. Other parents smack because they don't know how to say 'no'. They grin and bear it for as long as they can and then suddenly they explode – yelling, smacking and punishing. To escape this unexploded-bomb cycle you need to learn how to say what you want to say, when you want to say it. (Take a look at some of the ideas in Chapter 6 and Chapter 7 for suggestions about alternatives to smacking and ways to cope with our feelings.)

Our parents teach us how to behave by what they do and say to us from the moment we are born. These lessons, learnt so early, are extremely hard to unlearn, because they form part of the basic building blocks of what makes us, us. But although it is difficult, and sometimes painstakingly slow, it is not impossible to learn different ways to raise our children.

After the Storm

This is the most important moment of any tantrum. What you do after your toddler has finished shouting and screaming will determine, more than anything else, how many more tantrums you will have to bear. Each of the suggestions below will feel right some of the time. Some days, a tantrum will make us hopping mad and other days it will be a minor inconvenience. The suggestions below allow you to pitch your response to your feelings. The aim of any response is to say exactly what you feel, when you feel it, and still leave your toddler with her self-respect. When you say what you want to, there is nothing left for you to brood on. Within these boundaries, whatever you do after a tantrum is fine. The important thing is to make contact with your toddler again, so that she sees the radical difference between your lack of attention during the tantrum and your full attention afterwards.

Kiss and Make Up

The most successful post-tantrum activity is a really warm and loving hug. Research evidence suggests that when kids get a hug following a tantrum they tantrum less often and for less time. When you scoop your child up into your great big protective arms she doesn't just get a hug she also learns three important messages:

- I'm still here.
- I care about you even when you are awful.
- Even when you fall apart I can help you feel together again.

A hug lets your toddler know that although you gave her no attention when she was screaming and shouting you do still love her and appreciate how hard this growing up business is.

There are all sorts of different hugs that fit different times in life. (Personally, my favourite is just after story time when my kids are drifting off to sleep, and nine times out of ten so am I.) The post-tantrum hug works best if you can put yourself into it wholeheartedly. This doesn't mean that you have to be forgiving and accepting immediately, or that you have to be the kind and accommodating parent you see in a hundred advertisements.

Quite the contrary. There's still some straight talking to be done, because you don't want many more of these tantrums. No, by 'whole-heartedly' I mean bring everything to it that you've got. Your frustration, your anger, your sadness and disappointment, your embarrassment, your feelings of failure, your expectations and your love of your toddler. It's a tall order. But if there is one important time for you to be genuine, it's now.

You can do this in two ways:

1 The Silent Hug

Often a wise move when you can't make sense of all those feelings of frustration and anger, exhaustion and helplessness coursing through you, and you just know that if you said anything it would come out as mean and nasty. Tantrums wind you up, hugs can wind you down. All sorts of feelings can be expressed and left behind in a vigorous hug. A woman I know, called Jackie, says that when she feels that murder is the best option she throws her arms wide and gives her kids all-enveloping bear hugs complete with growls. She hasn't murdered anyone yet. But everyone in her family is well hugged.

2 The Reasonable Hug

This is for those times when you have either dealt with your frustration during the tantrum or are having a good day. The aim of this hug is to reason with your toddler. Try any or all of the following elements:

- Describe what set her off: 'You wanted to tell me that the cat was in the garden but I was busy on the phone.'
- Tell her what you want her to do next time: 'If you want to talk to me when I'm on the phone come and say "Excuse me" first and then wait while I ask the person on the phone to hang on a second.'
- Explain why she can't have your attention right now: 'When I'm on the phone, I have to talk and listen to daddy or Auntie Sue … so I can't hear what you are saying to me. The people on the phone are important to me so I want to give them all my attention.'
- Give her hope for the future: 'As soon as I put the phone down you are my most important person and I can give you all my attention.'
- Reject her tantrum: 'When you had the tantrum it was loud and scary for you, and I felt cross. The tantrum stopped us talking to each other. Tantrums are not OK. I don't want to see any more tantrums.'

But if this all seems too controlled and soft, and the anger and frustration that's still bubbling inside you won't let you give your toddler a 'no-holds-barred' cuddle then you need to deal with that anger first.

Wait until the tantrum is over, take your toddler to a quiet place and then let rip. Let your toddler know in no uncertain terms that:

- tantrums are unacceptable
- you are furious and disappointed with her for behaving like that
- you expect better of her next time
- she should go to her room for two minutes/say sorry/some other immediate punishment (a punishment delayed is a lesson lost)

It's OK to be cross with your child for putting you through the mill. Anger is not something that you should keep under wraps. Nice people do get angry. But keep to the point. You may remember all the other 27 times your toddler has made you embarrassed in public, but she doesn't. Dredging them up now just makes her miserable without giving her any way out. This is why it's better to say:

- 'I felt embarrassed when you threw yourself in front of the lady's trolley in the supermarket' rather than 'Why do you always have to show me up?'
- 'If you want some sweeties, ask please' rather than 'You're always whining on at me for something.'
- 'I think you should say sorry for the way you acted just now' rather than '... and you never say sorry.'

When you're cross with your toddler say (or shout) what you have to say clearly and directly:

- without running your toddler down, or calling her names
- without smacking her
- with as much force as you feel
- then forget it and move on

That way your message is clear and your toddler has a chance to put things right because she knows what you expect her to do. Life is too short for recriminations. Each tantrum needs to be dealt with at the time and then forgotten.

Once your toddler has been punished remember to have that cuddle. It's OK to be angry if you feel angry, but it's essential that you make loving contact with your toddler soon afterwards.

A Word About Anger

In some families anger is a big taboo. For children and adults living in such families anger can be extremely hard to express. In other families people blow their top, shout at each other and then hug. Things get very passionate, but everyone feels fine. How you are brought up affects how safe you feel in getting angry. If anger wasn't permitted in your family, or your parents weren't able to cope when you became angry, you may feel that you need to keep a tight rein on your angry feelings, or they will destroy you and possibly everyone around you too. Many parents who are scared of anger tend to put up with far too much from their children, and then suddenly they explode. It's a common pattern. Expressing any emotion takes practice. To get this practice when you're grown you may want to book yourself in for some counselling where it will be safe to get angry. Talk to your GP in the first instance.

Just one last thing before we leave the practical side of dealing with tantrums … The only thing that doesn't work once the tantrum is finished is bearing a grudge. If there's one thing that's worse than a tantrum, it's a sulk, and bearing a grudge teaches your child to sulk. People who sulk are almost impossible to live with. They haven't learnt how to ask directly for things they want so they are unable to accept direct requests or apologies from others. Nothing anyone does is right or good enough. Living with someone who sulks is exhausting.

So don't swop tantrums for sulks. Express those feelings then leave them behind.

6

How to Cope with the Way You Feel

Dealing with your own emotions when your toddler has a tantrum.

When Gavin's toddler, Alex, throws a tantrum in the supermarket he becomes flustered. Sometimes he asks lots of questions hoping to make him stop screaming: 'Alex, what's up? Did you want that toy? Do you need a wee?' At other times he pleads with Alex to stop. 'Oh Alex, stop sweetheart, it doesn't help. Please stop, Alex.' Neither works. Gavin's wife, Debbie, gets cross with Gavin, she knows that ignoring Alex works best. And that Gavin's obvious embarrassment just makes Alex worse.

But Debbie also knows that Gavin's reaction comes from his own childhood in which his mother ignored him until he was naughty and then yelled at him: 'Be quiet, what'll the neighbours think?' You can see why he's so anxious for Alex not to disturb the other people in the supermarket. Unfortunately, it's the same with happy sounds too. When Alex's cousins come to play they run upstairs like the proverbial herd of elephants. Here again, Debbie happily goes with the flow while Gavin leaps up and down the stairs endlessly urging them to be quieter. He acts rather like a big brother – warning them of impending doom, of the punishment of some greater power – but he never gets them to be quiet because he isn't firm. In this way, he goes on being the anxious little boy he was.

Childhood feelings are extremely potent. If we learn to be anxious, or feel we are clumsy, or feel that to be loved we have to cope on our own as children, then we often go on feeling the same way into adulthood when we have the opportunity to teach our kids all that we have learnt.

Accepting Our Own Feelings

Tantrums are emotional explosions for your toddler, but unfortunately they can also result in emotional explosions for adults: emotional explosions that can reverberate for hours. There is nothing wrong with feeling cross or frustrated, embarrassed or exhausted when your toddler tantrums – so long as you don't join in with the tantrum by shouting, screaming or slapping.

It's all too easy to use our feelings to excuse the way we deal with tantrums. 'I felt so angry I couldn't help myself.' 'I was so embarrassed I just exploded.' 'He just got me so mad, I ...' The truth is that feelings don't *make* us do anything at all. We, unlike our toddlers, have a choice about what we do. We can't help the way we feel but we can take responsibility for our actions. That is what we are trying to teach our toddlers. And before we can teach them, we have to learn it for ourselves. It is not an easy lesson.

We only give feelings the power to make us act in unhelpful ways when for one reason or another we don't look at them squarely. We have to be honest about how much of what we feel is to do with his bad behaviour when our toddler throws a wobbly and how much is to do with feelings we don't like to talk about too much, but which are being dredged up by his tantrums.

Toddler tantrums can leave us feeling:

- angry
- unable to cope
- shocked
- unable to bear staying with him

At times, for some parents, there is an unsettling sense of ambivalence when their toddler tantrums: they feel curiously excited but they also want to make him stop. Often, the feelings are more intense than any feelings we can remember having had, for years. Toddlers are incredibly frustrating so it's not surprising. But if it seems that these feelings will overpower you and drive you to do or say things you would regret, then you need to begin to look at them seriously, away from your child. Take stock of how you feel, and then talk about it with someone who is prepared to listen. Language is what ultimately saves your toddler from the grip of tantrums, and it can save you too.

Learning From Our Own Childhood

Some of the extremes of feeling that tantrums evoke may have been hidden inside us for years, possibly since childhood. We learn a lot from our parents and what we learn helps us to become the people we are. As children, we believed that our parents were perfect – and that whatever they did, whatever they said, they were always right and they always loved us. As children, we did everything we could to hold on to that illusion. Some of us cast ourselves as the bad guys whenever mum or dad did something unreasonable or insensitive, while others blamed someone else. Imaginary friends or brothers and sisters were very useful here. Some of us locked away the bad feelings we had because they seemed too awful to face.

It can be useful to simply acknowledge how we felt when our parents didn't seem to understand us, like us or even love us or when their every word seemed to be a criticism.

Imagine the scene. You, as a two-year-old have just fallen over and grazed your knee, and you are crying hard. Now look at the chart below. What might your mum or dad say, what do you feel and how does it change you?

Mum or Dad Says:	You Might Feel:	Next Time You Might:
I told you not to run	Misunderstood, cross, foolish	Lie to avoid the blame Be frightened to run
Oh, look at your trousers	Unimportant (your trousers are more important than your pain)	Try to cope on your own, but feel lonely
Not again	Helpless (they must expect you to fall)	Be anxious so that you are more likely to fall
You're all right, stop whingeing	Unloved (they don't care that you're hurt)	Cry more loudly or give up crying when you're hurt
Oh-ho! Sounds like you have a sore knee there. Let's have a look	Understood. It's OK to cry when I'm hurt	Cry if hurt, and find someone to help

Do you recognize any of these feelings? Think about times when you felt that your parents didn't understand you and times when you felt that they did – what was it that they said or did, and how did you feel? Were there times when they labelled you as clumsy, or stupid, clever, or pretty. Were those labels difficult to bear even when they were supposedly nice?

Parenting Ourselves

When we were little, feelings had the power to make us shrink or come out fighting. As adults, we can look back at the child we once were and feel sorrow and love for our small selves, accepting our anger, fright,

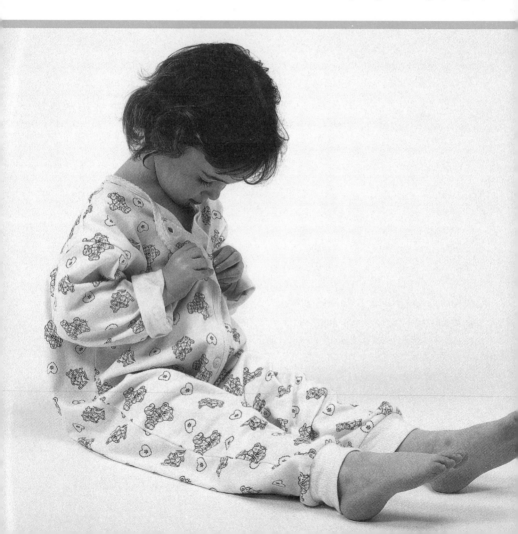

confusion and loneliness. As adults, we can parent that child as we would have wanted to be parented – with warmth and honesty, openness and secure boundaries. Such quiet thoughts can help us to soften our attitudes, firstly to ourselves, and secondly to our own toddler's tantrums.

Knowing that we can be the sort of parent the child inside us would have loved gives us the strength to contain our toddler's emotional extremes without feeling threatened. We can do for our toddlers what we are now learning to do for ourselves.

This is not an easy or a quick process. For many people it is impossible to do it alone. If your own childhood has left you feeling threatened or confused you may find that counselling helps. Contact your GP and they can advise you.

Stress

Of course, not all of our reactions have their roots in our childhood. Some of the time temporary stresses leave us scrubbed raw by feelings, which we then try to avoid.

When we are under stress most of us try to cope by shutting out some of the intensely emotional reactions. In some ways, this is a good idea. If your mother dies or your child is seriously ill, you may need to ignore how you feel for a while in order to cope with the practicalities.

But if this emotional shutdown goes on for long it can cause problems. We can become:

- unable to ever let any of it out, perhaps even long after the original problem has resolved itself
- so busy coping that we forget how to live
- unable to recognize the need for feelings at all

Of course, it's not just we who suffer when we learn to hide our feelings. As parents this sort of holding in can affect our toddlers in two different ways. Either we:

- Find it difficult to allow our toddlers to express anything fully:
  Millie: 'Oh no, the paint has spilled all over my lovely picture.'
  Mum: 'It's only a small spill, don't make such a fuss.'

or we:

- Let our children express those extremes of emotion that we can't express ourselves:
  Becky: 'I don't want to go home, I'm going to stay here.'
  Dad: 'Perhaps grandma would let us stay until bedtime.' (I want to stay here too but I don't feel I can ask for myself.)

Most people who are hiding from their feelings do both at one time or another.

When we sometimes refuse to allow our toddlers to express how they feel and at other times secretly find relief in their tantrums, we can see that we have become inconsistent. And inconsistency leads to tantrums.

The solution lies in unbuttoning that sad or angry person inside us, and making it safe for him to express himself. That way we no longer have to rely on our toddlers to help us cope, but can take responsibility for the way we feel, and responsibility for how we behave.

The important point is not to deny your feelings, but to be aware that you can handle them – whatever they are. Everyone feels anxious, angry, frustrated and a hundred other emotions but, with practice, you can come to accept those feelings and still think creatively when you hit the inevitable problems of parenting. Telling yourself that you can manage precisely *because* you accept your own and your toddler's feelings, can help. Which brings us to the second part of cracking tantrums.

Focus on a Solution

Once you have acknowledged how you really feel about your toddler's tantrums, you can think more clearly about what you want to do about them. How you are going to solve your problem. Chapter 5 has lots of practical suggestions. Tantrums are a wonderful opportunity to teach your toddler what you have just taught yourself: that strong emotions are a natural part of life which can be weathered, and through which we can grow. You can do it.

In Your Toddler's Shoes

Try putting yourself in your toddler's shoes. He's trying to be more grown-up, more independent, than he's ever been before. If you were trying to do something difficult, something you had never attempted before, something that stretched your abilities to the full, how would you feel if your partner, seeing you struggling, said:

- 'There's no need to scream.'
- 'Here, let me do it for goodness sake.'
- 'Why do you always make such a fuss?'
- 'You're just being silly.'
- 'It's easy.'

Or even:

- 'Shut up', accompanied by a well-aimed slap.

If you're anything like me, you'd probably feel one or more of these things:

- misunderstood
- even more cross
- resentful
- helpless
- stupid

And if you'd been slapped – outraged, shocked, vengeful and scared. But if your partner really felt for you, and was big enough to prevent his or her own frustration leaking out, she or he might say something like:

- 'That's really difficult, isn't it.'
- 'Is there anything I can do?'
- 'I could do with a break myself, do you want to take five minutes?'
- 'I don't know if it would work for you but sometimes I find it helps if I …'

So why does this feel so different? Some of the reasons could be:

- your partner understands what you are going through
- your partner treats you as though you are a reasonable human being
- your partner isn't blaming you for your reaction
- your partner sounds as if he's in control of his own emotions, which is reassuring
- your partner isn't trying to take over, or belittle you
- your partner isn't annoyed with you

- your partner leaves the responsibility with you
- it feels OK to give up or to continue, whatever you choose

Of course, no one can be this saintly all the time, parents of toddlers perhaps the least of all. But if, on a good day, we can remember what it feels like to be a toddler, and react in kinder ways, our children will tantrum less and love us more openly.

It's Not Just Toddlers who Tantrum

Just one final thought before we leave this subject of adult emotions. We all have times when everything feels too much. Thoughts like:

- 'I could just walk out now.'
- 'Why do I have to do all this?'
- 'I know I can't afford it but I'm going to buy it anyway.'
- 'I know I've had enough but I'm going to have one more drink/cake.'
- 'If I start shouting now I'll never stop.'

All of these are adult equivalents to the heel-drumming, blood-curdling screaming of your toddler. 'I can't cope with this responsibility, I didn't want it in the first place, let someone else do it, it's not my fault, help, help, help.'

But these times come and go, and with an arm around your shoulder and an empathetic ear, they pass more easily. Your toddler will benefit from the same loving approach.

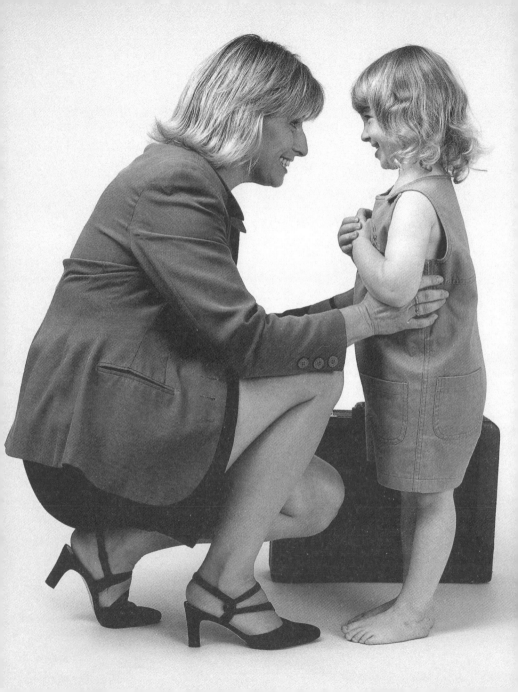

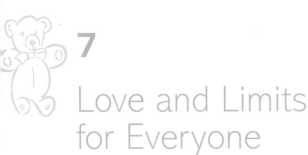

7
Love and Limits
for Everyone

It's tough being a parent, whatever the age of your children. But being the parent of a toddler is one of the toughest.

The other day, I led a discussion about toddlers. 'What,' I asked the assembled parents, 'does it feel like to be the mum or dad of a toddler?' It wasn't all pretty. There were shouts of 'exhausted', 'like I can't get it right', 'frustrated', 'really happy and then suddenly really cross', 'confused', 'out of control', 'like walking on thin ice', 'like a meanie when I have to yell'.

Toddlers stretch you in every way – emotionally, physically, intellectually and socially. But most importantly they stretch your belief in yourself. So that most caring parents begin to ask 'What am I doing wrong?' It's an unsettling time.

Meanwhile, back at the group, we agreed that it could be a time of extremes. 'OK, so much for the grown-ups.' I said 'What do you think your toddler feels?' This time the list seemed strangely familiar. 'Exhausted', 'like he can't get it right', 'frustrated', 'really happy and then suddenly really cross', 'confused', 'out of control', 'like she's walking on thin ice', 'like a meanie when she yells'.

Ring any bells? The fact is that toddlers and their parents often feel the same. And this, strangely, may be helpful. Once you realize that you and your toddler are somersaulting through the same emotional hoops, you can begin to appreciate what she is going through. You may not like the way she expresses it, but you can empathize with the feelings.

But why are these emotions so much more in evidence during the toddler years than they are at any other time (except perhaps adolescence)? The answer is that toddlerhood is a transition. Your toddler is in transition between being a baby and being a child. She is in the process of leaving behind a babyhood in which she accepted things at face value, and reaching out for a childhood in which she will be surrounded by things that she can understand. Two islands of calm. But from her present position very little seems certain, least of all her image of herself and her sense of where she fits in. And when she loses her precarious sense of who she is then she's likely to collapse into a tantrum. The same process of dramatic and agonizing self-redefinition happens in the teenage years, when adolescents try out all sorts of personalities (stroppy, cheerful, leader, queen of cool) before they find one with which they feel comfortable.

It's an emotional time for you, because frankly, life with a megalomaniac, self-centred, but unselfconscious, scientist who has a 12-minute concentration span on a good day, can be frustrating.

What's So Special About Toddlers?

Between 18 months and three years (give or take a month or two either way) toddlers start to build up a picture of who they are, and how they fit into their family and the wider world. What you say to your toddler and do or don't do for her now will have dramatic and long-lasting consequences for her:

- personality
- ability to cope with strong emotions
- self-esteem
- social skills

- attitude to authority
- independence

If your toddler feels that she can rely on you to help her through frustrations, without babying her, and that you still love her even when she's ranting and raving, but you like it better when she's not, you will have a stronger relationship in the years to come.

In a minute, we'll look at the sorts of things we can do to help our toddlers grow into happy, responsible children. But just before we do, let's just have one last look at the way that parents and toddlers feel. It's clear that parents and toddlers often feel the same negative emotions. They can, and often do, share the same positive emotions too.

The parents in the discussion group also said that they and their toddlers were loved and fascinated, protective and entertaining, excited and happy.

If you can find ways of being with your toddler that make you feel happy, the chances are that your toddler will feel that happiness too. And if you can treat your toddler in ways that make her feel good about herself, the chances are you'll feel good about yourself too. Feelings are contagious. You might as well work on the good ones.

Everyone is Special

The first and most fundamental job you have to do as the parent of a toddler who is ultimately to grow into a happy and responsible adult, is to: Make sure your toddler feels special.

Everyone needs to feel special. Parents, children, even grandparents. It's a basic human need. Up there with food and shelter, water and freedom. Feeling special means that we are loved just because we exist, because we are unique, not because we are funny, or cute, pretty or cheeky, but just because we exist. Without the warmth that comes with feeling special we can't grow, we can't look outside ourselves and welcome others in, and we find it much, much harder to make anyone else feel special.

You can help your toddler to feel special in lots of ways:

- spend time with your toddler
- give your toddler your undivided attention when she seems to want it, as often as you can (two minutes now is always better than half an hour later on)
- listen and respond to your toddler
- try to understand your toddler
- accept your toddler in all her emotional turmoil, and frantic busyness
- tell your toddler how special she is to you, just because she is who she is
- when you have to tell her off, be sure to make up again afterwards – whatever you do, don't hold a grudge

Time for Yourself

But what's sauce for the goose is sauce for the gander. In other words you need to feel special too. So try some of the same techniques on yourself:

- spend time on your own, and don't allow any interruptions
- acknowledge and accept your own feelings
- try to understand yourself
- accept that you're not perfect but …
- … you're still special
- don't punish yourself when you lose your cool. You are not the worst parent in the world

A Word to Those who Find it Hard to be Good to Themselves

No matter how much you do for your kids there will always be more you could have done. But good parents are in the business of raising clever, brave and kind kids who like themselves and respect and love others, not tyrants who expect everything on a plate and for whom nothing is ever enough.

There have to be limits to what you do for your toddler and limits to what you allow them to do to you. Everyone's limits will be different – I've known parents who positively love it when their toddler runs in at six in the morning for a cuddle. They feel that the lost hour's sleep is worth it for the warm little body and the gorgeous smile. While others have a 'no one out of bed until seven' rule. Fine. Some parents cook fish fingers, sausages *and* pizza for tea reasoning that, at least this way, everyone eats. While others cook just the one meal and operate the 'take it or leave it' rule. No problem.

The point is that if you're happy with the way you do things you will have a largely contented toddler. But if you feel guilty when you don't do what your toddler wants, and harassed or put upon when you do, then your limits are in the wrong place for you. Guilt, like plastic bags, should be kept away from babies and toddlers at all times. Attention that comes wrapped up in guilt can just as easily smother and choke a baby as a plastic bag. Toddlers know when you really want to be with them. Give your time freely, not because you are trying to make up for something. If you're feeling guilty sit down and talk through what you are doing with your partner or another sympathetic listener.

Then set those limits at a point where you feel good – at a level where you still have the chance to be you and your toddler has the chance to be herself. This way, at least you get some time to yourself.

What this means is that you give your toddler your hundred per cent attention whenever you can but you also take 10 or 15 minutes off (at least once a day) just to be you. No demands, no whining, no 'just this one thing', no nothing. Make sure your toddler is safe and happy and shut yourself into the kitchen, or the garden or your bedroom and do whatever you like (but anyone caught ironing or tidying will be shot at dawn).

Maybe you could read the paper, have a coffee, chat on the phone or just sit quietly, it doesn't actually matter. But whatever it is make sure you revel in it, you deserve it. You are special and you need to celebrate that fact.

But over and above that, you also need to plan for longer time away. A weekend with your partner or on your own can re-establish the sense of yourself that living with a toddler erodes. A little bit of what you fancy does you good. In time away, you can go at your own pace, meeting no one's demands but your own. It is a vital part of parenting, especially the parenting of a toddler, that you remember who you are, so that you can have a clearer sense of who your toddler is as well.

Time to Be and Time to Do

But it's harder still, when life is packed, to justify doing nothing. Yet all of us, no matter how busy we are (in fact, especially if we feel busy), need to stop regularly and do nothing, on our own. It's an amazingly difficult thing to do. Stop what you are doing. Do nothing. Be alone.

Usually, when we sit still our minds carry on buzzing. I remember the first time I tried it I noticed the chipped paint around the door, I remembered that I hadn't got any milk, I wondered if my son was OK at playgroup, I remembered that I hadn't been in to see my neighbour for a few days and so on and so on … In fact, I beat myself up for doing nothing while all those important things were left undone. But I persevered, and gradually the 'to do' list disappeared and I found myself mentally browsing through the day, and making connections with other days, other feelings and other people. Now, I also stop off en route to places and take in the scenery, or in the middle of washing up, stop and look out of the window for a couple of minutes. In that space I know I grow as a person.

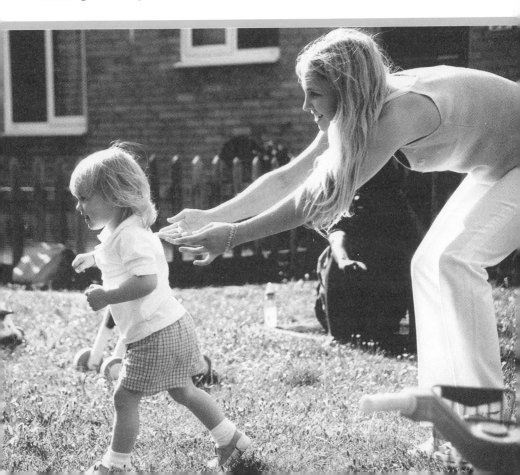

Most of our lives are spent doing things. It's how we define ourselves. 'Hello, I'm Jane, I'm a teacher', 'Hello, my name's Tim, I work at the jeweller's', 'Hi, I'm Molly, I'm a full-time mum, chauffeur, cook, cleaner ...' But we need to feel special just because we are alive too. Being still lets this happen.

Being still has great knock-on benefits for your children too. Once you learn to handle the silence without needing to fill it you can:

- listen better
- stand back from your children's demands
- not have to have the last word
- not feel that you have to have the solution immediately
- let go of the control
- give yourself time to think
- allow your children to be bored
- allow your children to be sad
- allow your children to express all sorts of other negative emotions
- allow a solution to come to your children

Being still is a great habit to cultivate when you are caring for a toddler – toddlers are frantically busy people and sometimes it seems that the only way to escape from their demands is to become busy ourselves. But no adult ever beat a toddler at that game. Being still is the antidote to busyness. Being still brings a balance to your life.

Being still is important for everyone, but it's vitally important for parents who didn't feel special as children. Parents who don't feel special need to learn how to grab this feeling for themselves before they can foster it in their children. Growing up allows us the opportunity to parent ourselves as we would have liked. Show yourself how much you are appreciated by giving yourself some time.

Children who don't feel special often end up as adults who are intensely competitive, or who drive themselves (and others around them) extremely hard. People who never sit down, whose houses are immaculate, or who make you feel guilty or inadequate by the amount they do, are sometimes struggling to prove that they are special. But all this activity is never enough – it's never able to replace the emptiness they feel when they stop. Far better to stop and face the emptiness, no matter how scary, because ultimately liking ourselves is the only way to great parenting.

Your kids don't just *deserve* a mum and dad who take the time to feel good about themselves and life – they *need* a mum and dad who take time out as well.

Limits

The second thing that you need to do to help your toddler grow up happy and considerate leads on from this. Toddlers are not just learning about themselves in isolation, they are learning how they fit into the wider world. And the best help that you can give your toddler in this is to: Set and stick to fair and consistent limits.

Again, you can do this in many different ways:

- devise rules about eating, sleeping, touching dangerous things, playing with others and so on
- have the same rules wherever you are – at granny's, in the park, at a friend's house
- stick to routines so your toddler knows what to expect
- limit the sort of behaviour you will accept from your toddler, for example no hitting or biting and no tantrumming or sulking
- limit the sort of reactions you make to your toddler, for example no smacking, no tantrumming, no sulking, no grinning and bearing it

- limit the time you give to your toddler – that is, insist on some for yourself
- but never limit her emotions or yours, what you feel is what you feel

You need to start limiting what your toddler can do and what she can expect of you because, at this age, toddlers have no self-control and will go on making demands of you all day and all night if you let them.

A toddler playing within firm and consistent limits may often be angry or frustrated and she will sometimes tantrum, but limits that are fair (and it is important to make sure that your limits are fair) are like a protective arm around her shoulder – they reassure her that someone cares enough about her to say 'no'.

Sam uses the tried and tested count-to-three routine:

> When Rachel is behaving unacceptably – kicking, a tantrum, not co-operating, and so on – I give a warning before I allow myself to get really cross. I say "I am going to count to three and then I am going to do X" (where X is always something really specific such as take the toy away). I then count slowly to three – none of this two and a half business! Usually by the time I am mentally at two and a half the behaviour has ceased. I only rarely have to carry out my threat, but always do it if necessary.
>
> **Sam, mother of Rachel, four**

When you look your toddler in the eye, raise your voice just a tad, and speak firmly, she feels secure and loved. She knows that she will be OK, because no matter how much she rants and raves you won't let her spoil things, endanger herself, or upset or hurt anyone else either. Little by little she becomes a touch more mature, a little more able to govern her own flimsy and ever-changing desires. She grows sure that she can handle the parts of life that you insist on her doing (sitting down at mealtimes, saying 'hello' to adult friends) and that she can do without the bits that you refuse to allow her (staying up one more hour, playing outside in the rain).

Love and Limits

If you only make your child feel special but don't give her limits she will become a tyrant – a tyrant that you will slowly but surely come to dislike. If you only limit her behaviour without showing her that you think she is great you will be the tyrant, and later she may find it hard to remember why she thought she loved you. Either one on their own doesn't work. Your toddler needs to feel that she is special and to know that there are limits to her behaviour and to yours. These are great lessons for life.

If your toddler is to grow up to be:

- a warm, compassionate and fun-loving child who has a firm sense of herself
- a child who isn't afraid to stand up for what she needs

she will need parents who are:

- warm, compassionate and fun-loving adults who feel good about themselves
- not afraid to stand up for what they need, and what their toddler needs

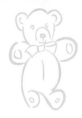

8

How to Help Your Toddler Grow Up

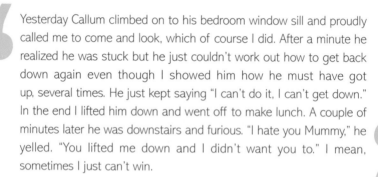

Yesterday Callum climbed on to his bedroom window sill and proudly called me to come and look, which of course I did. After a minute he realized he was stuck but he just couldn't work out how to get back down again even though I showed him how he must have got up, several times. He just kept saying "I can't do it, I can't get down." In the end I lifted him down and went off to make lunch. A couple of minutes later he was downstairs and furious. "I hate you Mummy," he yelled. "You lifted me down and I didn't want you to." I mean, sometimes I just can't win.

Jo, mother of Callum, three

It's impossible to get it right with toddlers all the time. In fact, you may not believe it, but it's your job to fail now and again. Good parents get it wrong now and again. So long as they feel that they are loved, toddlers grow up (just a little) every time we give them our best shot and miss. Just like adolescents, toddlers need someone to love and to hate in order to make it to the next stage of their lives. If they can't fight with you, they can't win through. In the next few pages we'll look at the issues that are big news for your toddler in his journey into childhood and consider what we can do to keep him on track.

In Chapter 7, we looked at the basic principles of all good parenting – love and limits. In this chapter, we will consider the specifics. How, precisely, do you make sure that the love and limits you give your toddler are the best they can have?

Fostering Independence

George Bernard Shaw once said 'Marriage is popular because it combines the maximum of temptation with the maximum of opportunity.' It's a bit like that with toddlers. Now that they've left babyhood behind them toddlers can see the potential in a great many new adventures – pouring bubble bath into the loo, bringing their sandcastle into the house to show you, taking a bite from each of the little cakes laid out for tea – and, given their rapidly improving physical skills and their lack of inhibitions, they will try all these and many, many more.

Some of the time, your toddler will love the fact that he can do it – dress herself, 'read' a book, climb the climbing frame – but at other times, like when he meets new people, or has to stay in unfamiliar places without you, or even for no particular reason that you can see, he will want you to help him a little bit more than you have been.

Life is not a straight line. We don't start at the beginning and go on, ever on, until we reach the end. On the way, there are hills and valleys, detours and dead ends and a lot of roundabouts that take ages to get off, because we just can't see the right way to go. At each stage of development and on into our adult lives we all need to circle a bit around problems before we feel confident enough to move on. The problem toddlers are circling is independence.

If you force him to move on – to act independently – when he doesn't feel able to, you may scare him. On the other hand if you insist on doing things for him to save time or mess or energy he may feel smothered and frustrated. It's not always easy to see what to do for the best.

Most of us want our kids to grow up confident, capable and caring. If they are going to end up like this we need to show them how. It's best to start when they are young.

The DAD Plan

For confident, capable and caring kids try the DAD plan. (Actually, just between you and me, it works just as well for mums!)

First: Describe the problem
Secondly: Accept the feelings behind it
Thirdly: Devise a solution

With preverbal toddlers you will have to do most of the talking.

Esme (18 months) is struggling to dress herself, but the Velcro strip on her shoes keeps sticking where she doesn't want it to, and it is making her mad. Finally she screams. Sarah, her mum, comes over.

- First, she describes the problem: 'Those Velcro bits are getting all over the place aren't they?'
- Next, she accepts the feelings behind it: 'Little things like that can make you go crazy.'
- Finally, she devises a solution: 'How about if you practise with the shoes off first?'

But as your toddler grows older the DAD plan becomes more of a joint effort. Take Jamie:

Jamie (aged three) is off to a party. It's supposed to be fun, but Jamie is worried because his best friend Robert isn't going. Margaret, his mum, comes to sit with Jamie.

'What's the problem?' she asks.

'I don't want to go on my own.'

'So, you don't want to go because Robert isn't going.'

(They've defined the problem.)

'Uh-huh.'

'And how does that make you feel?'

'No one will play with me, I'll be on my own.'

'Oh, so you're feeling anxious that you won't have anyone to play with.'

'Yes.'

'Mmm, that sounds difficult. I get nervous before parties too – they're kind of exciting but scary too.'

(They've accepted the feelings.)

Margaret goes on: 'What shall we do about it?'

'Stay here.'

'OK, that's one way round it. Do you have any other suggestions?'

'You could stay at the party with me.'

'Uh-huh. Anything else … No …? Mind if I suggest something? Maybe we could call up Rory and ask if he wants to go to the party with us – that way you would have someone to go in with.'

'Yes, call Rory. And you stay as well … just for a minute though, because it's really a children's party, and they won't have enough cake for you.'

(They've devised a solution.)

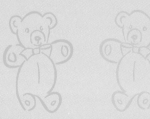
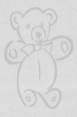

Notice that:

- Margaret gives Jamie the chance to find his own solutions, but when he's stuck she offers an alternative. Her alternative answers the fear of being alone that Jamie has already talked about. If she had said 'Oh, you'll be fine' and left him to get on with it at the party he would have been anxious, and angry with his mum for misunderstanding.
- Margaret doesn't rule out any of Jamie's suggestions immediately. Later, if Jamie hangs on to his ideas, Margaret can rule out the ones that wouldn't feel right for her and he can rule out the ones that don't feel right for him. (In fact, Jamie does this at the end when he asks his mum not to stay too long.)

The DAD plan lets your toddler see:

- the problem clearly
- that it's OK to need you
- that no matter how intensely he feels things, he can cope

Love and Hate

Everyone, your toddler included, is more likely to say 'I love you' when things are going well and they feel good about themselves. For toddlers in particular, this feel-good factor comes when it suddenly strikes them afresh that they are comfortable with the level of independence they have achieved. On the other hand, toddlers say 'I hate you' when they feel babied and do not want to be, or when they feel pushed to be more independent than they can manage. It's your toddler's way of showing you that you do not understand what he needs. It's painful, for both of you, but it is not all bad.

It's in the gap between his expression of some need and you meeting that need that your toddler will grow. When you get it wrong, your toddler feels frustrated, but he also learns that this frustration doesn't destroy him. It's an important lesson for life. A toddler who is never frustrated, never learns that he can cope. A toddler who can't cope with frustration in small doses will be unable to handle life's ordinary frustrations when he is older.

If your toddler does tell you he hates you, try not to take it as his final word. Within a surprisingly short time your toddler will turn himself sunny-side up again and you will be flavour of the minute.

Loving parents don't meet all their toddler's demands immediately.

Allowing Sadness

Toddlers' tears can be difficult to bear. Every parent wants to make them stop. But toddlers, like the rest of us, need to be allowed to be sad. If this sounds crazy, just think what sort of message you give your toddler when you ask him to stop crying, before you've even tried to understand how he feels. He may feel that:

- he was somehow wrong to cry
- the thing he was crying for was unimportant
- you won't love him unless he's happy

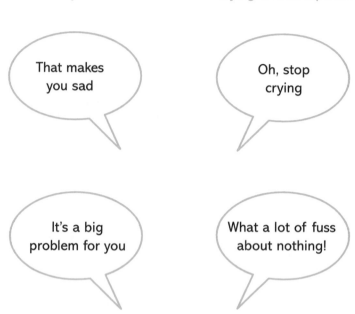

That makes you sad

Oh, stop crying

It's a big problem for you

What a lot of fuss about nothing!

So stick with your toddler when life is giving him a hard time, listen to his howling and try to describe what he must be feeling. He may not stop crying quickly this time, but he will learn how to understand and talk about his feelings for the future. In the long run he'll be able to talk rather than scream, and what's more he'll know that you cared about him when he was sad. Toddlers grow up happier and calmer if we listen to, and take seriously, the apparently little things on the way.

It's easy to feel embarrassed or angry when our toddlers make a lot of noise, especially in public, but parenting is a long-term job with long-term goals. The more seriously we take our toddler's fears and concerns now, the more easily he'll leave them behind:

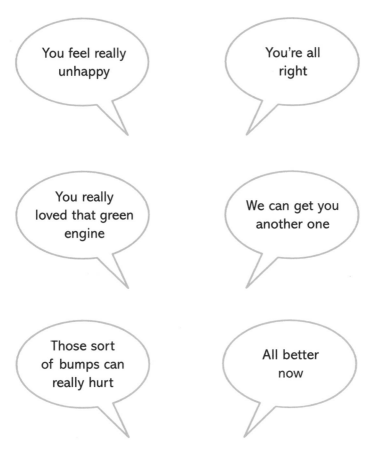

You feel really
unhappy

You're all
right

You really
loved that green
engine

We can get you
another one

Those sort
of bumps can
really hurt

All better
now

Being allowed to be sad gives your toddler the chance to:

- see that his emotions won't kill him
- find his own solutions

Resist the temptation to wave a magic wand and make everything right.

If we don't allow our toddlers to feel some sadness, they can't experience the intensity of real happiness, and if you can't have happiness then you've lost something precious.

Helping our kids to feel good about themselves and yet still feel their emotions deeply takes not just time but emotional energy too – prepare to work out.

Saying 'No'

The toddler years can feel very negative. Many a toddler's favourite word is 'no'. Even, funnily enough, when they actually want to say 'yes', many toddlers still say 'no' just to keep their hand in. Your toddler says 'no' because it's the only way he knows of gaining control. He is learning to take control but he isn't there yet.

A toddler's favourite word may be 'no' but a very wise mother once pointed out to me that a toddler's second-favourite word is 'Mummy'. Those two words are the battle for independence in a nutshell.

On the other hand many parents find they are saying 'no' more often than they like. They, too, are struggling to keep control over a toddler who is intent on going his own way. So, how can love and limits help here?

When Your Toddler Says 'No'

You can love and limit your toddler by taking a minute to understand why he is saying 'no'. Maybe:

- you have pushed him to do something he can't manage
- you have held him back from something he wanted to do
- you interrupted him
- he's angry
- he's embarrassed …

I could go on, but I'm sure you can fill in the gaps.

If you are at fault, do something about it. Otherwise, the trick is not to pay too much attention to his 'no' unless he is about to do something dangerous or unkind, in which case you will need to lift and remove him. You'll need to decide which things it's worth insisting on.

When You Want to Say 'No'

Try to turn your 'no' into a 'yes' or a 'later' if you can. Get down on your child's level and be warm and compassionate. What does he really want by:

- pulling your trousers while you're washing up?
- insisting that he wear his coat and wellies on the hottest day of the year?
- demanding that you play with him when you've just sat down to feed the baby?

You may want to say 'no' to all of these:

- 'No. Don't pull my trousers.'
- 'No, you can't wear your wellies today, take them off.'
- 'No, I can't play with you, I have to feed the baby.'

But an outright 'no' puts you at loggerheads with your toddler. Better to show that you can understand his point of view by turning those 'no's into a 'yes' or a 'later' if you can.

Tell him in words that you understand what he wants and then tell him what you are prepared to do about it:

- 'I can see you are in a hurry, let me just dry my hands and we can talk.' (Which is 'a tiny bit later'.)

Or:

- 'You want me to be with you don't you. Here, let's do the washing-up together.' (Which is a 'yes'.)
- 'You love those clothes don't you. I think you're going to be hot, but OK.' (Which is a 'yes' – after all, he'll probably take them off when he gets hot.)

Or:

- 'You love those clothes, I know that. If you put on your shorts and T-shirt or your skirt and top before I count to 10, you can change back again when we get home from the park.' (Which is a 'later', with the added bonus of a choice, which is all-important to toddlers.)
- 'I'd love to play with you. Let's just see if the baby will finish her feed and sleep, and then we can play for longer.' (Which gets you and your toddler on the same 'grown-up' side.)

Or:

- 'Yes, I'd love to play with you. I was just going to feed the baby. Maybe she can wait. I'll tell you what, why don't *you* tell *me* when you think the baby is hungry.' (Which gives your toddler the chance to be in control, and to show how caring he can be.)

Toddlers have to learn how to wait just like everyone else. But they learn best when the lesson is repeated for short spells and often. Of course, sometimes you do have to say 'no', but try to keep these to a minimum and stay calm.

Making Excuses and Blaming Others

Most of us recognize that our toddlers are less than perfect. But sometimes we act in ways that make them feel we blame them for it. Sighing heavily or acting the martyr can become a pattern. And sentences that begin with the words 'Do you think just once you could ...' or 'Not again ...' make our toddlers feel that:

- they have done wrong
- we expected them to do wrong
- we blame them for it
- there is no obvious way to do right

It's an easy pattern to slip into in the toddler years because of the frequency with which we seem to have to ask our toddlers to stop something or to start doing something else:

'Oh, William, look what you've done now – videos all over the floor.' 'I've got enough to do without you spilling drink on the floor.' 'Big boys don't do that.')

Next time you feel ready to blame, stop and consider:

- What's the real problem here?
- What can I do about it, right now?
- How can I stop it happening again?

Take Pete. His three-year-old, Midge, has deliberately walked through the puddles with her sandals on, in spite of being asked not to, and is now wet and miserable.

Pete bends down to Midge's height and looks her straight in the eye.

- He states the real problem: 'Oh-ho, it looks like you have wet feet from those puddles.'
- He says what they can do: 'Let's see if we can shake some of that water out, and then go home the quick way.'
- He (tries to) stop it happening again: Later on, when Midge is warm and dry, Pete talks about different shoes for different fun and he and Midge agree that sandals are best for jumping and boots for splashing.

Pete doesn't blame Midge. She already feels miserable, and the walk home will be long enough without a lecture. He focuses on what he can do, which is to go home. Later, he makes sure that it doesn't happen again (or at least not too often).

On the other hand, we sometimes get into the habit of finding excuses for our toddler's behaviour so that we don't have to change our perception of them as being perfect.

'Jessica only hit Greg because he got too close and she didn't like it.'

'Nick just gets so excited; it's a real shame when the other children don't let him go first.'

'Will you two big boys please let Ryan play. He's only messing things up because he feels left out.'

Better to get down to your toddler's level and:

- describe what happened
- show you understand why
- state the rule
- suggest two alternatives (remember, a choice gives him a chance to feel good)

'Jessica, you hit Greg. You didn't like it when he came too close, did you. But nobody hits anyone here. Next time you could walk away or say "Move away." '

'Nick, you pushed in to go first. You were really excited about the slide. But nobody pushes in here. Next time, wait in line or choose something else to play on.'

'Ryan, you messed up Nathan and Steve's game. You wanted someone to play with. But no one's allowed to mess up someone else's stuff. Next time, ask them if you can play, or find a game of your own to play.'

Older toddlers can answer for themselves. All you need to do is prompt them for the answers:

'What did you do?' 'I pushed in.'
'Why?' 'I wanted a go.'

'What's the rule about that?' 'No one's allowed to push in.'
'OK, what could you have done?' 'Go on the swing.'

If we don't acknowledge that our toddlers are, like us, both good and bad, kind and mean, they won't feel comfortable with all the various bits of their personalities. We do our toddlers no favours when we see only their faults or only their virtues. Kids who feel that they are all good or all bad are unhappy or deluded kids.

Allowing Failure – a Better Kind of Success

Superparents are a pain to live with and so too are children who feel they have to be perfect in order to meet their parents' expectations. Here are some of the techniques that children who feel that they can never be good enough adopt:

- competitiveness
- blaming others
- lying
- pretending that they were going to do that next
- nervousness
- bullying
- becoming a victim
- acting

It's a sad list. If you recognize three or more of these characteristics in your toddler, now is a good time to make yourself a little less perfect. Once you feel comfortable with the new 'good enough' you, you can let your toddler off the hook now and again.

Like a lot of us, Lindsey's a bit of a perfectionist. But recently she's started to change. Now, when something she's been struggling with goes wrong she doesn't throw up her hands in horror or stomp around the house yelling at innocent bystanders like her husband, the kids and the dog. These days, Lindsey uses the powerful image of a hot-air balloon to carry all her imperfections away. Lindsey's balloon is green, but you choose your own colour.

She finds herself a quiet corner somewhere, closes her eyes and imagines herself packing the basket under the balloon with whatever it is that she doesn't feel is perfect – a cake, an argument with her husband, the kitchen wall she painted or a chapter she has edited – and then she lets it go. She lets it go, and the balloon floats up into the blue sky, lighter than air, taking the weight of her troubles away and making light of them until they are nothing more than a speck in the distance, bobbing small and insignificant. One small trouble in a vast heaven of pale blue. Then she opens her eyes and feels content with what she has achieved. Perfect it is not, but it is a lot better than it was before, and she can be proud of that.

Try it.

Saying Sorry

One of the best ways to avoid being perfect is to say 'sorry'. It's just as true for parents as it is for toddlers. Our toddlers need to hear us say 'sorry' when we get things wrong. And if you can't think of the last time you got anything wrong maybe you should ask your toddler. He will know.

It's a funny thing, saying sorry. The more we get into the habit the less we actually need to say it. Saying 'sorry' makes it OK to go on trying to be good and failing. Not being able to say 'sorry' means we have to hide our failures or blame someone else. At least when we try to be good, we have more chance to succeed.

All of us screw up from time to time – it's what makes us human. If you never admit to putting a step wrong, there's no way that you can expect your child to either.

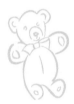

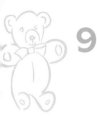

9

Beyond Toddlers

Tantrums Don't Last Forever

Luckily for all of us, most toddlers outgrow tantrums. There are six main reasons:

- They learn to use words rather than to scream (although frustration can still tie their tongues on occasion).
- They learn to see things from someone else's point of view (especially where the other person is familiar).
- They learn from experience – and the average three- or four-year-old has a lot more of that than the average 18-month-old.
- Toddlers' ability to concentrate, their memory and attention to detail, improves. All of this means that waiting for just a minute isn't the impossible request it once was.
- They have a better understanding as well as a lot more experience with two important ideas: that one thing can represent another and that you can sort things into groups. This means that if their brother accidentally drinks their juice it isn't the end of the world – because there's more juice where that came from and there are other cups too.
- They learn to manage on their own a little and they don't need you quite so much as they did. It doesn't matter so much if things don't stay the same because change won't destroy them.

With your loving, time-giving, firm and consistent approach all of these things are easier to learn. By the time they are three or four, most toddlers have come to terms with some pretty extreme emotions: they have learnt the best way to ask for help when they need it, and the limits of the behaviour you will accept. They know where they stand and, most of the time, they feel comfortable in that position. Knowing more clearly who they are, and who you are as well, they feel better equipped to handle the next challenge of life ... but that's another book.

Good Books
and Other Resources

Steve Biddulph (1998) *The Secret of Happy Children* London: Thorsons
Steve Biddulph with Shaaron Biddulph (1999) *More Secrets of Happy Children* London: Thorsons
Adele Faber and Elaine Mazlish (1980) *How to Talk so Kids Will Listen and Listen so Kids Will Talk* New York: Avon Books
Dr Christopher Green (1998) *Toddler Taming* London: Vermilion
Penelope Leach (1997) *Your Baby and Child* London: Penguin
Asha Phillips (1999) *Saying 'No': Why It's Important for You and Your Child* London: Faber and Faber
Michael and Terri Quinn (1995) *From Pram to Primary School* Newry: Family Caring Trust
D.W. Winnicott (1991) *The Child, the Family and the Outside World* London: Penguin

Telephone Support:

Parentline-plus 0808 800 2222
A free confidential helpline service for anyone in a parenting role.

Useful Internet Sites:

www.kidsource.com   www.relate.org.uk
www.babycentre.co.uk   www.parentplus.org.uk

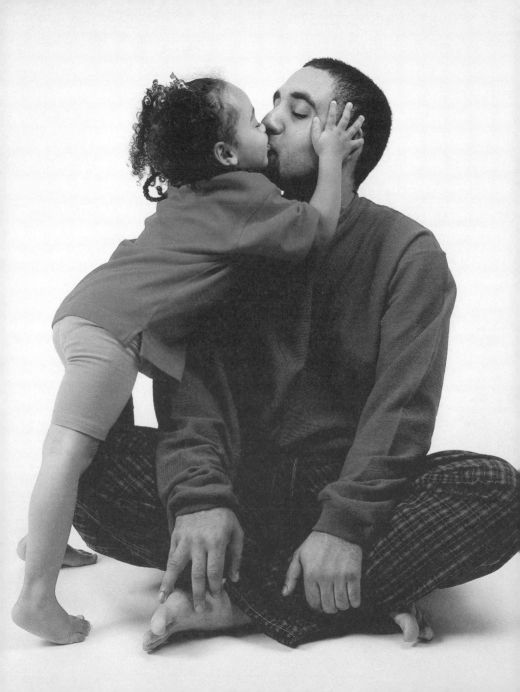

About the
National Childbirth Trust

Run by parents, for parents, the National Childbirth Trust is a self-help charity organization with 400 branches across the UK. There's bound to be a local branch near you, running:

- childbirth classes
- breastfeeding counselling
- new baby groups
- open house get-togethers
- support for dads
- working-parents' groups
- sales of nearly-new baby clothes and equipment

– as well as loads of events where you can meet and make friends with other people going through the same changes.

- To find the contact details of your local branch, ring the NCT Enquiries Line: 0870 444 8707.
- To get support with feeding your baby, ring the NCT Breastfeeding Line: 0870 444 8708. Any day, 8am to 10pm.
- To find answers to pregnancy queries, ring the Enquiries Line or log on to: www.nctpregnancyandbabycare.com

- To buy excellent baby goods, maternity bras, toys and gifts, call 0141 636 0600 or look at: www.nctms.co.uk
- To join the NCT, just call 0870 990 8040 with a credit card.

You don't have to become a member to enjoy the services and support of the National Childbirth Trust. It's open to everyone. We do encourage people to join the charity because it helps fund our work – supporting all parents.

When you become an NCT member and join your local group, you'll get a regular neighbourhood newsletter (a guide to your area aimed at new parents) and you'll also receive NCT's *New Generation* – our mailed-out members' magazine that takes an in-depth look at all issues of interest to new parents.

'The NCT support network is second to none. It's very reassuring and comforting.'

The National Childbirth Trust wants all parents to have an experience of pregnancy, birth and early parenthood that enriches their lives and gives them confidence in being a parent.

National Childbirth Trust
Alexandra House
Oldham Terrace
London W3 6NH
Tel: 0870 770 3236
Fax: 0870 770 3237

Index

Other titles in the series:

Help Your Baby to Sleep

Penney Hames

Practical steps to help you establish a routine with your baby that will look after his or her needs – and yours, too.

185 x 150 mm
£6.99
0-00-713605-6

Breastfeeding for Beginners

Caroline Deacon

This guide will provide you with all the help you need to begin breastfeeding and continue successfully.

185 x 150 mm
£6.99
0-00-713608-0

First Foods and Weaning

Ravinder Lilly

Ravinder Lilly answers all your questions about weaning your baby and how to provide a good variety of the right foods using simple recipes.

185 x 150 mm
£6.99
0-00-713607-2

Successful Potty Training

Heather Welford

Helps you spot when your child is ready to move out of nappies and decide on the right method for you both. Includes tips for when you are out and about.

185 x 150 mm
£6.99
0-00-713606-4